A POSITIVE APPROACH
TO CANCER

A Positive Approach
to Cancer

Patricia Gauden

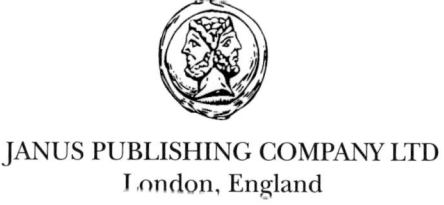

JANUS PUBLISHING COMPANY LTD
London, England

First published in Great Britain 2011
by Janus Publishing Company Ltd,
105–107 Gloucester Place,
London W1U 6BY

www.januspublishing.co.uk

British Library Cataloguing-in-Publication Data
A catalogue record for this book is available from the British Library

ISBN 978-1-85756-747-2

Cover Design and all photographs supplied by Mr D. V. Davenport ARCP

Printed and bound in India

Contents

Dedication

Dedicated to all the cancer patients, and their families and friends, that I have had the privilege to have known over the last thirty years – they know who they are … Their generosity allowed me to walk alongside them on their unique and individual cancer journeys.

Their courage, vulnerability and strength are to be applauded, as cancer affected every part of their lives and almost every day they were presented with new hurdles to be faced. I hope in some small way I have been able to use their experience of cancer to help others. This book carries their voice!

A crisis event often explodes the illusion that anchors our lives.

Robert Veninga, *Bag of Jewels*

Foreword

A person exists on many levels, all of which are equally real and important. Health is a matter of balancing the whole – your mind, body and spirit – resulting in perfect health and completeness.

A definition of holistic medicine is continued use of conventional medicine together with complementary medicine, psychotherapy and health education.

The mind, body and spirit approach to cancer is designed to facilitate the development of your own self-healing through empowerment, to regain control over your life, reverse the stress caused by a cancer diagnosis and to see how cancer can give you a life-changing opportunity. You will be in a position to make healthy choices and changes by uncovering and accessing your own needs, by exploring and understanding how your mind affects your body and by learning and discovering your inner strength. This approach works in parallel with medicine, whose aim is to begin to treat and then repair your body following a diagnosis.

A diagnosis of cancer can be devastating to all concerned and you will no doubt remember the details surrounding it clearly. Each patient's reaction to cancer is different and unique to them. For some, the shock of the word 'cancer' is too much and they just want to get out of the hospital or clinic as soon as possible; others cry uncontrollably or get angry. All of these demonstrate normal emotional reactions and the need to express them, which is healthy.

For those who care for a person with cancer, it is often very hard to watch someone you love cry uncontrollably or become angry or withdrawn or, alternatively, even deny what is happening. It is also hard for the carers not to take this personally. Each person has to face this in their own way and then find their own way of dealing with it. Whatever decisions they make, it is their choice and their family need to respect and support that choice.

If the decision a person reaches is with other people in mind or, indeed, made by other people then the balancing of the mind, body and spirit of that individual will never be achieved. They will be doing one thing, but thinking and feeling another. Incongruity takes over and communication, which is so important at this time, becomes very difficult, as the patient's commitment to their own treatment and recovery will be lacking.

Introduction

In 1977, as a newly qualified nurse, a gentleman called Len was admitted with a bowel obstruction and I was asked to prepare him for theatre. Later that day, I arrived in the post-operative recovery room to escort Len back to the ward and was told that the cancer was inoperable. The surgeon met with Len's wife and family that evening and said that there was nothing that he could do, because the cancer had spread. He then advised the family to take Len home.

Because the consultant had had no contact with Len after surgery, Len had assumed that this meant that everything was all right and that the cancer had been removed as planned. His wife and children now had the burden of either telling Len that there was nothing more that could be done or just keeping it a secret.

In a split second, Len and his family's life had changed forever. For me, the words, 'Sorry, there is nothing I can do' remained with me and I felt that there must have been at least something that could have been done. I made a momentous decision on that day to specialise in cancer care, otherwise known as oncology, and become better prepared to deliver all the options of care that cancer patients could and should be offered.

It is now thirty years later and over the years I have had the opportunity to work in some of the best specialist cancer hospitals in the UK, as well as working in the community, patient's homes, cancer centres and hospices. Over the years, I have experienced major changes in cancer care, not only in relation to surgery, radiotherapy and chemotherapy but in early diagnosis, in genetics, in the way patients now access cancer care and in prognostic longevity, which now accounts for many patients living with cancer for many years.

The organisation of cancer services has changed for the better. Clinical trials have produced many new cytotoxic drugs and we now have new understanding of the structure of our DNA, which is helping scientists to unravel our genetic make-up in relation to cancer.

Thankfully, patients are no longer willing to accept that 'nothing can be done'. They are proactive in finding out what is available on the

Internet, not just nationally but internationally as well. As a result, they are now able to identify support agencies and obtain information on specific cancers, cancer diets, geographical information regarding specialist cancer centres and the option of where they would like to be treated.

The biggest step forward for me has been from the general public, who are now willing to talk about cancer, to find out about preventative cancer care and to seek early diagnosis. They are also now able to discuss various treatment options and to gather factual evidence, which then allows them to make an informed decision about their own treatment options.

Now, in the twenty-first century, new challenges face us. These days, many patients are treated and they remain disease free for ten years or more and oncologists would tentatively call this a cure. However, it is also an emerging fact that many patients are being diagnosed with a second primary cancer often unconnected to their original cancer and therefore many need to go through all the trauma of diagnosis and treatment for a second time round, because their life style had not changed at all.

Almost all families now know of someone within their family and circle of friends who has or has had cancer. How could this happen? Clearly, we don't have all the answers yet, as the cause of cancer is multifactorial. One major factor is lifestyle and it is this issue that I explore within this book.

Cancer care for me is not only about the specific skills of surgeons, radiotherapists and oncologists, at the point of diagnosis and treatment, but also the continued support for as long as the patient needs it. Individuals facing cancer have mind, body and spirit needs that are not always fully addressed in modern oncology units. It is one thing to say 'ring us if you have any problems' as the patient leaves hospital to go home, but it is quite a different experience when the patient is at home and no longer has that support around them. When they return home, it is then that the reality of living with cancer really begins.

This book seeks to draw on the countless experiences I have listened to over the years, from patients and their families and friends to clinical staff and volunteers. It also explores a holistic life philosophy, not just for your cancer journey but for living with or without cancer. It is divided into three main sections, mind, body and spirit, containing patients' tips and solutions, together with pages for reflection, positive quotations and uplifting photos. It offers new ways to perceive and interpret life's challenges and demonstrates how your choices make a real difference in your life. It is also about changing your lifestyle to reduce your risk of developing another cancer.

Pick up the book whenever you feel the need to. It is not a book to be read from cover to cover. Dip in and out, take out of it what you need, what is relevant for you now, and come back to it later. It is a book which will raise many questions, allowing you to refer back to it at any time. Remember, if you change only one thing about your lifestyle, it will be your first step towards making a real difference in your life.

Reflection

Take a moment to reflect.

Throughout the book, you will be reminded to take a moment to reflect. This will allow you time to pause and reflect on the picture or words, or the section you have just read. Or it may ask you questions on which you may like to ponder and reflect on your response.

The art of self-discovery is about being able to reflect on the decisions you make every day, all of which influence your mind, body and spirit, and ultimately your wellness. We all live in a state of imbalance. The secret is being aware of this and then taking positive steps to correct it.

I am sure you have often asked yourself many of the following questions, since you or a loved one was diagnosed with cancer:

- what did I do to deserve this?

- how could this happen to me?

- what is the deeper meaning of this illness?

- what is cancer telling me about the way I live?

- what can I do to change the impact that cancer is having on us, as individuals, as a community, as a country or globally?

Learning that you have a serious illness, like cancer, can offer you a life-changing opportunity, allowing you to take time to reflect on your state of mind and body and your spiritual approach to life and to recognise where there may be an imbalance. It may be about:

- choosing to take 'me time' each day

- taking time each day to meditate

- connecting each day with nature's rhythms

- seeing the beauty in everything

- treating your body with love, compassion and reverence, appreciating its remarkable resilience in the face of adversity

- making each day count

You can explore some of these within the pages of the book that remind you to reflect or you may want to share your thoughts with someone you love. For some, a separate journal for reflection may be a better choice, rather than writing in this book; it may be that you write in it each day or as and when – the choice is yours! Reflection in silence helps to quieten the mind and you will soon see a difference, especially if you approach it with an open mind.

At times of emotional turmoil or when faced with difficult decisions, it is often in the silence of the night, or the stillness of the early morning, that many of your feelings rise up and overwhelm you. If alone at this time, using a reflective journal allows you to safely explore your feelings through words, or a drawing or a poem.

Listen to your inner voice of intuition; it is guiding you. Stop to reflect on what gives meaning to your life today. Turn a negative thought into a positive action, take back control over your life and discover just what it is that is important to you now. From today, anything is possible. Allow forgiveness and unconditional love to walk beside you, to drive away your fears.

Reflect on life's beauty, the first snowdrops, a child's love and spontaneity, a loving touch, a thoughtful word, a gesture, a smile, the beauty of the sunrise or the sunset, something that made you laugh. What was it you did today that made all the difference? What precious memory will you take from today to sustain you tomorrow? Your reflective journal is not intended to be either judgemental or to induce feelings of inadequacy. It is an opportunity to reflect one day at a time or one week at a time.

Take a moment to reflect.

The secret of making something work in your life is, first of all, the deep desire to make it work: then the faith and belief that it can work. Then to hold that clear definite vision in your consciousness and see it working out step by step, without one thought of doubt or disbelief.

Eileen Caddy, *Begin It Now*

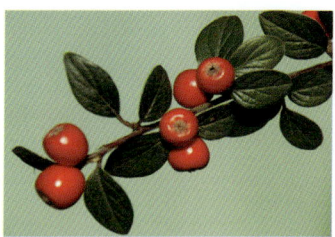

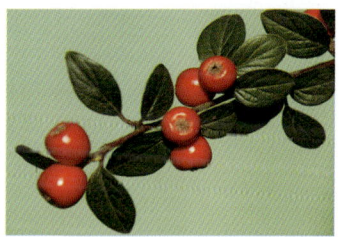

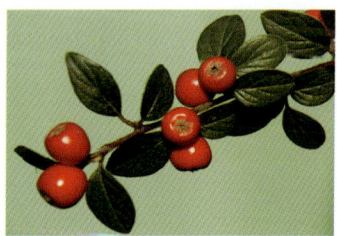

Cancer and the Mind

It is good to have an end to journey toward;
but it is the journey that matters in the end.

Ursula K Leguin, *Taking Time To Just Be*

Mind Matters

The mind's ability to think, wonder and reflect elevates human beings from other members of the animal world. Stillness of thought and the absence of harmful addiction allow the positive energy of the mind to flow freely and release energy for creativity and learning, to reach beyond apathy and face life's challenges. Assessing the energy balance of your mind helps you to highlight important areas of mental stress and anxiety in your life, caused by the cancer or the cancer treatment. There are five factors that determine the balance of your mind's energy: happiness, learning, empathy, self-esteem and beliefs and values.

Happiness:

Happiness allows you to embrace life fully with an open heart. It is a source of inner contentment and harmony. You express happiness spontaneously through fun and laughter and it expands when you have someone or something to love and care for; something to hope for and something to create.

Learning:

Learning builds wisdom and character. It allows you to broaden your knowledge, develop new skills and reach your own potential. Learning about yourself is possibly your greatest achievement in life as it feeds your enquiring mind and adds to your understanding of your life's purpose.

Empathy:

Empathy means accepting and honouring the unique needs of other people, with sensitivity and sincerity. We can give of ourselves by being there for another person and by listening without judgement. For some, giving is more comfortable than receiving or vice versa. For energy flow, giving and receiving both need to be balanced.

Self-esteem:

Your self-esteem reflects your feelings of personal worthiness and your willingness to care and value yourself. Building self-esteem is achieved through listening to your own intuition, integrity and instincts and being proactive in caring for yourself. A high self-esteem facilitates the full enjoyment of life, which will, in time of need, give you inner confidence to face challenges and difficulties. It is inspired by faith in your inner self and it liberates you from fear. You feel worthy of life and you feel connected to the world.

Beliefs and Values:

The voice of your conscience helps you to distinguish between right and wrong. It means applying your soul's wisdom to your daily life and ever striving to attain your highest good. Your values allow you to incorporate what is the truth for you in everyday life. If you compromise your beliefs, this may cause disharmony and an imbalance of your energy, which will manifest itself in 'what you think', 'how you feel' and your 'subsequent behaviour'. Individuals need to know that what they do is valued. They need to give themselves permission to meet their own body, mind and spirit needs in order to feel cared for.

Your first and most valuable relationship is with yourself. If you are not comfortable with that relationship, you are unlikely to feel comfortable in any others. Take some time to reflect on who you put first:

- If you do not value yourself, why should anyone else?

- How often do you do something that someone else wants you to do, not what you want to do?

- How often do you do something just for you?

- Do you feel internal conflict because you are not being true to yourself?

Take a moment to reflect: do you prefer to give, rather than receive? What can you do to enjoy receiving rather than giving?

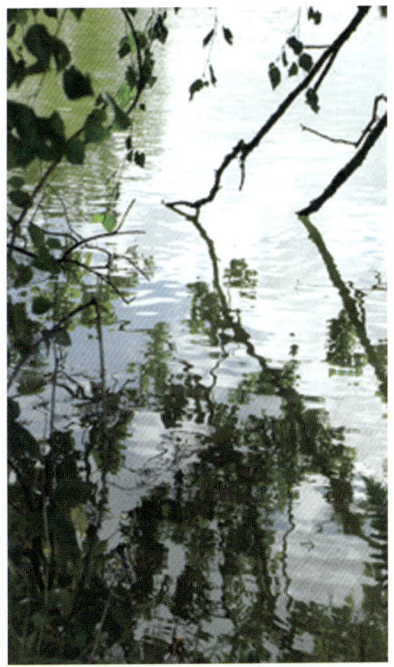

You are in physical existence to learn and understand that your energy, translated into feelings, thoughts and emotions, causes all experience. There are no exceptions.

Seth, *Bag of Jewels*

Stress and the Mind

Stress is a word we now use or read about daily. Much is written on the negative effects of stress in many areas of our lives. A diagnosis of cancer causes stress for all concerned: the patient, their family and their friends. A certain level of stress, however, is natural, beneficial and even essential to life. Your body's sympathetic nervous system provides you with an effective stress response to enable you in times of danger to 'fight' it or 'flee' from it. It puts your body systems on alert, concentrating blood flow, oxygen and energy to where it is most needed.

In contrast, your parasympathetic nervous system reverses the alert response, muscle tension is released, your heart rate slows, your blood sugar levels decrease and your breathing rate returns to normal.

Today, high expectations, together with our need for instant solutions and gratification, make stress an inevitable part of our everyday life. Stress is created within us by our perceptions and images. You experience the symptoms of stress in your mind and body when you go beyond your natural level of coping. This occurs when there is either a perceived or an actual threat to your mind or body.

You may find a stressful situation overwhelming, leading to changes in your feelings, thoughts and behaviour. It may help you to approach the situation using the following three-stage process:

What kind of threat is this?	Challenge
What can be done about it?	Optimistic choices
What coping strategies help?	Reduce Stress

Therefore:

The challenge	Cancer
The optimistic choice	Specialist treatment
Stress management	Relaxation/imagery

Coping is:

■ proactive

- the critical link between stressful life events and how you adapt to them

- about drawing on your own hidden resources

- about remembering to breathe

The best way to control fear is to face it and then explore and access one of your own coping strategies to overcome the fear.

Patient experience:

> After I was diagnosed with cancer, I found that the people around me no longer told me how they were or asked me how I was. They were afraid of raising the subject of cancer with me, in case it upset me, and sadly this also stopped me from expressing how I was, in case I upset them.
>
> One weekend, when all the family were at home, we sat down and explored this issue. I introduced a blackboard system to hang in the kitchen, which allowed everyone each day to score how they were feeling from 1–10. Today, I score 8 – it's a good day, a day full of opportunities!

Patient experience:

> For most of my life, I have wanted everything to be perfect. I orchestrated key times in our family's life to ensure we portrayed a sense of perfection in all areas of our lives.
>
> When I was told I had cancer I suddenly realised just how much energy and stress the need to be perfect had taken from me each day. Cancer allowed me to be just me, with all my idiosyncrasies. No more role-playing, no more pretence. Now, the most important thing in my life is my family and friends, who were all relieved when I stopped the need to be perfect!

Patient experience:

> John had spent all his life working towards a perfect retirement, which was now twelve months away. He and his wife had no children, they had paid off the mortgage and

they were planning to move to Spain, to enjoy their retirement. They had booked a world cruise for a month after his official retirement. Instead of taking expensive holidays each year, they had been content to save for the future.

All of those plans were shattered when he was diagnosed with lung cancer. He refused treatment and he and his wife brought the cruise forward. The last time I saw him, he said, 'Don't wait to do the things you want to in life, live those dreams now!'

Look to this Day!
For it is life, the very Life of Life.
In its brief course lie all the
Varieties and Realities of your Existence.
The Bliss of Growth,
The Glory of Action,
The Splendour of Beauty;
For Yesterday is but a Dream,
And To-morrow is only a Vision;
But To-day well lived makes
Every Yesterday a Dream of Happiness,
And every Tomorrow a Vision of Hope.
Look well therefore to this Day!
Such is the Salutation of the Dawn!

extract from the Sanskrit,
Taking Time To Just Be

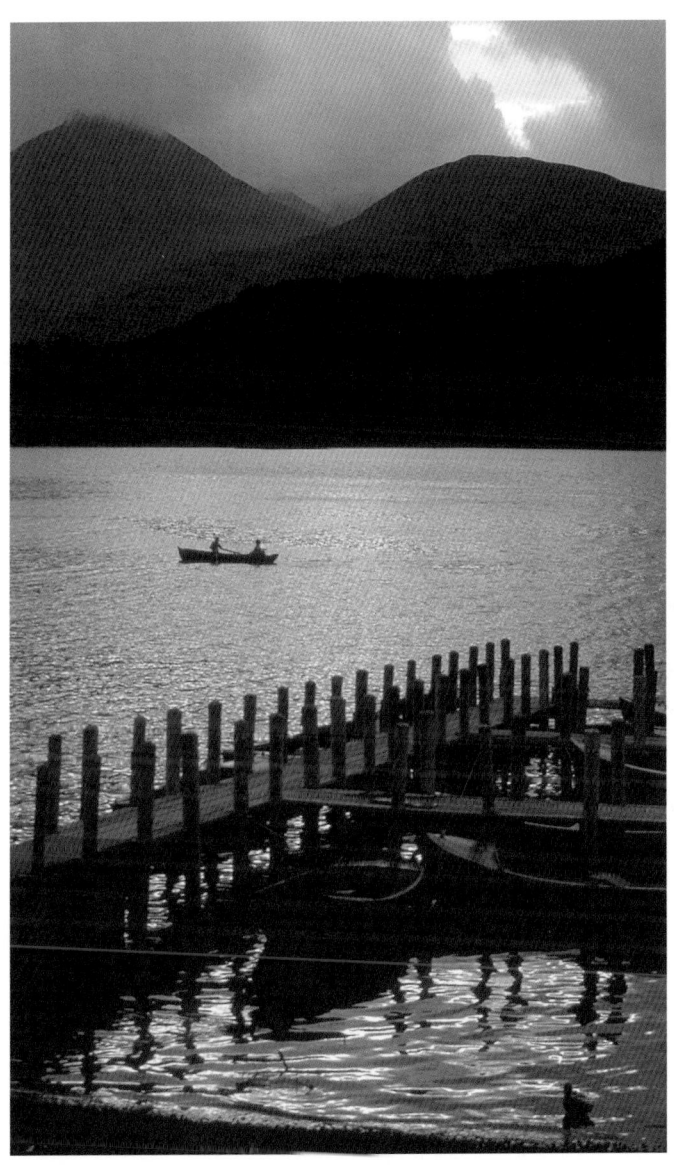

If You Listen

Stop for a moment during the day
And let the sun bathe your face.
Take a second or two to listen to the music
of the laughter of your children as they play.
Go to the river bank and listen to the sound
of the water. The chirping of the birds, and
the blowing of the wind.
It is the world around us that speaks to you.
That will inspire you. If you listen hard enough,
you will find the voice within yourself, and the
ability and the power to make a difference.

Erin Brockovich, *Take It From Me: Life's a Struggle But You
Can Win, Taking Time To Just Be*

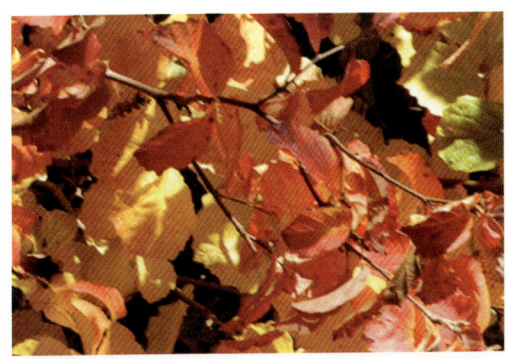

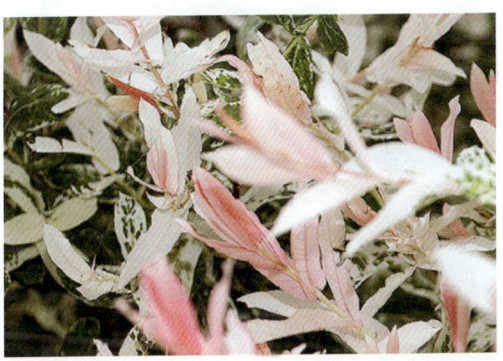

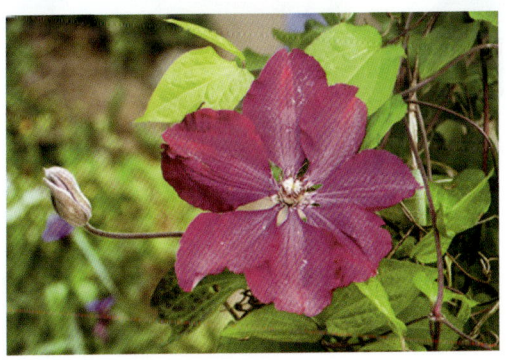

Take a moment to reflect: can you recall past stresses? How did you cope with them?

What would you attempt to do if you knew you could not fail?

Dr Robert H. Shuller, *Begin It Now*

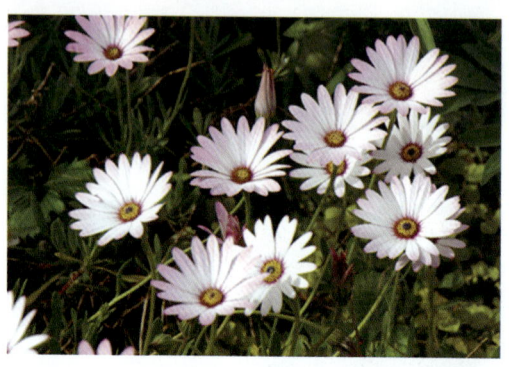

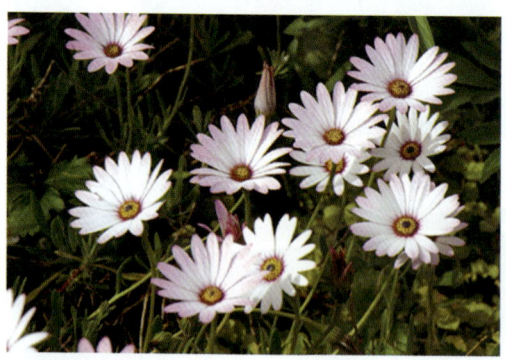

Things turn out the best for the people who make the best out of the way things turn out.

Art Linkletter, *Begin It Now*

Fighting Spirit

The cornerstone of your inner mental strength and fighting spirit is influenced by your personal values and beliefs. The value and respect you have for yourself is the fuel of your fighting spirit. Your personal beliefs sustain your mental strength and allow you to be true to yourself and to follow your own instincts and intuition.

On good days, your inner strength helps you to live life in the here and now. On days that are not so good, you may experience conflict between what you feel and what you think, and as a result you give 'confused' or 'mixed messages' to yourself and others. On days such as these ask yourself:

- What is making me feel like this?

- How are my thoughts affecting my feelings and behaviour?

- Listen to your inner voice and the message it is giving you. Is it self-supporting, reaffirming and encouraging in a positive way or is it self-oppressing and destructive, causing you doubt and confusion? Try applying the following awareness exercise when you are facing difficult situations:

Past situation:

Think of a situation in your recent past that you found stressful. Close your eyes and picture the scene. Remember the event and replay it in your mind, from the beginning to the end. Can you remember your thoughts and feelings as you went through the event? What was your intuition telling you?

Future situation:

Can you think of a situation in the future that may cause you anxiety and stress? Close your eyes and picture the scene. Go through the situation from start and finish. How does it make you think and feel? How could you have handled the situation differently if you needed to face it again?

Before the event:

A positive approach will help you to cope well with each situation; your inner voice will say something like, 'Stay calm; you can cope with this situation if you think it through.'

During the event:

Keep reassuring yourself that you can cope this time, as you now know what you want to achieve.

After the event:

Your positive inner voice will say, 'Well done; you handled that well.' Now think about how you feel. What are your emotions and thoughts? Did it help you through the situation? If it did then try to apply it when you face other stresses in your life. Remember:

Before: identify the stressor. What is it?

During: identify what you want to achieve.

After: identify what you will say to yourself after the event. How will you feel?

Noticing your thoughts will allow you to begin the process of change by:

- refusing to say anything negative
- refusing to think anything negative
- avoiding friends who dwell on the negative
- letting negative thoughts go
- switching the negative button off!

Positive imagery can change how you perceive life as it is today. How you can use this imagery is covered in the next section.

The following pages contain photographs of the four seasons and thoughts that we associate with them respectively. Can you imagine the seasons? How do they make you feel? What words do you associate with spring, summer, autumn and winter? Are they life-enhancing and positive? Does a specific season have negative connotations for you and if so, how can you change that?

Every day is a gift, open it, celebrate it, enjoy it.

Stuart and Linda MacFarlane,
Taking Time to Just Be

Take a moment to reflect:

Imagine a winter season –

The air blows cold

Frost skims the ponds

The trees are white and frosty

The air is crisp

The earth is cold and hard

The days are long and dark

Animals hibernate

The earth appears to sleep

All is quiet and still

Bulbs are growing

Roots are searching

The first green shoot of a snowdrop as it pushes itself up towards the light.

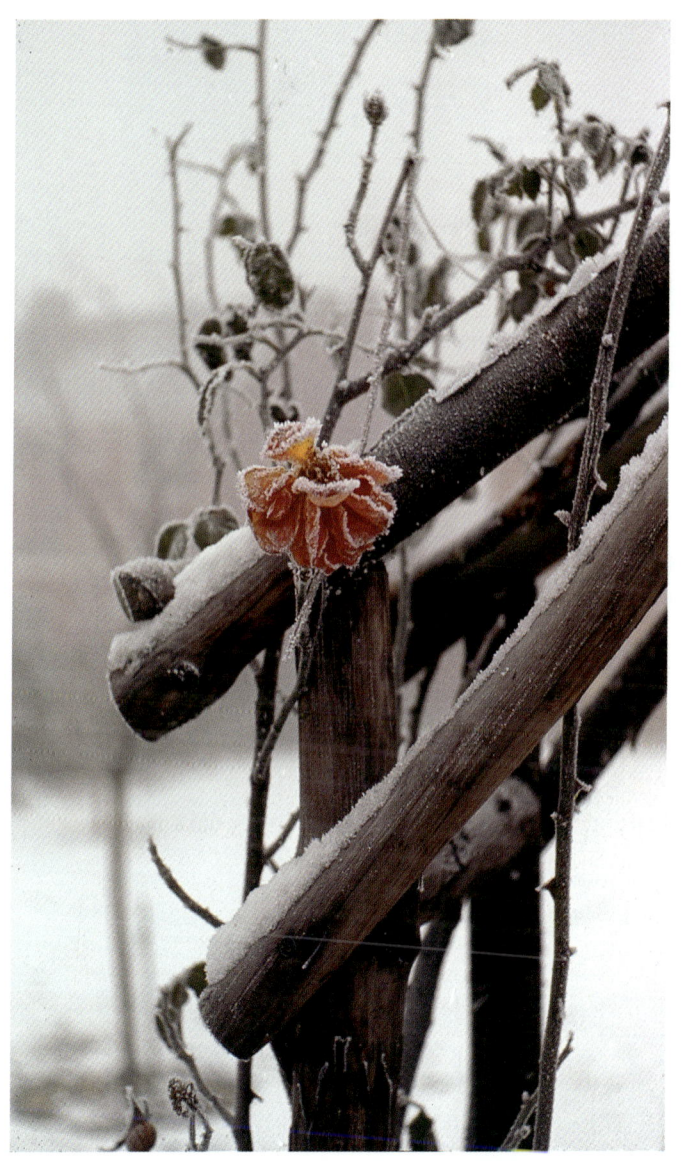

Take a moment to reflect:

Imagine a spring season –

The ground warms up

Daffodils herald the spring

The days lighten up

The earth starts to prepare for growth

Spring flowers bring with them the message of renewal, hope, life

Birds are nesting

Frogs are spawning

The blossom is forming

We long to be released from the long, dark days

Our bodies need the sunshine.

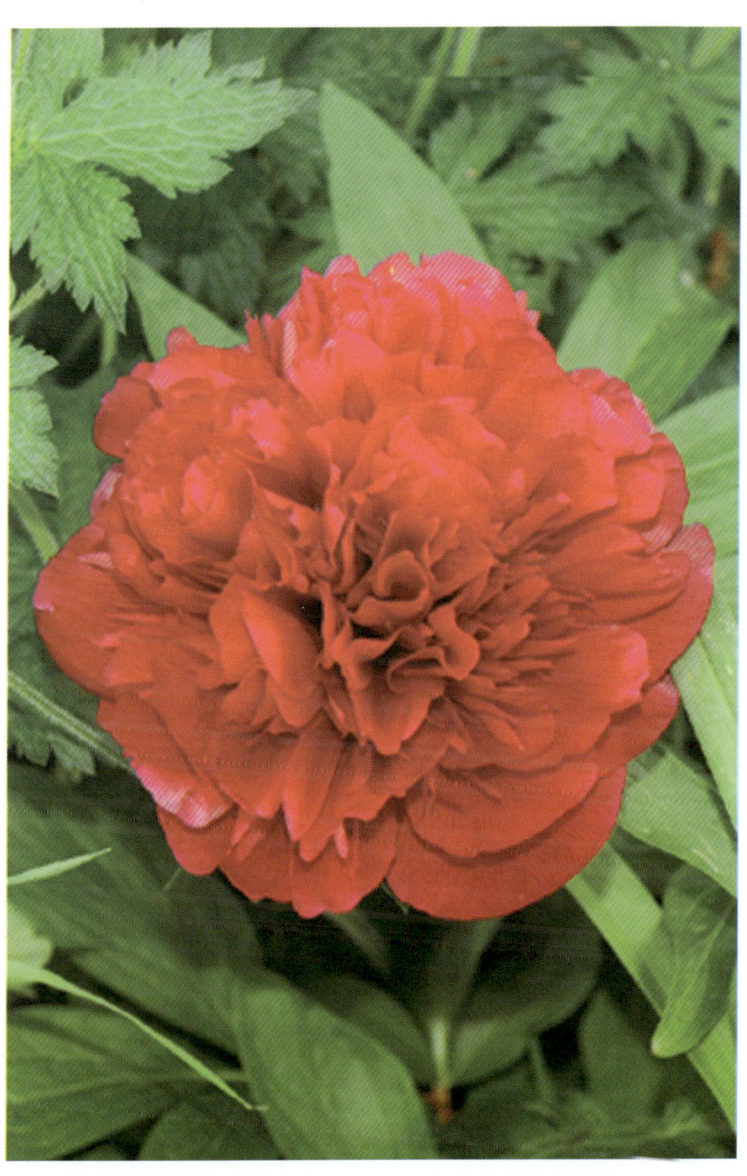

Take a moment to reflect:

Imagine a summer season –

A summer cottage garden

A pond full of water lilies

Borders full of peonies and roses

The perfume of wallflowers in the air

Lavender creating a safe haven for bees and butterflies

The heady scent of honeysuckle

Bowls of strawberries, raspberries and blackberries

The warmth of the sun creating total relaxation

Humming bees, singing birds

The hammock rocking slowly in the afternoon sun.

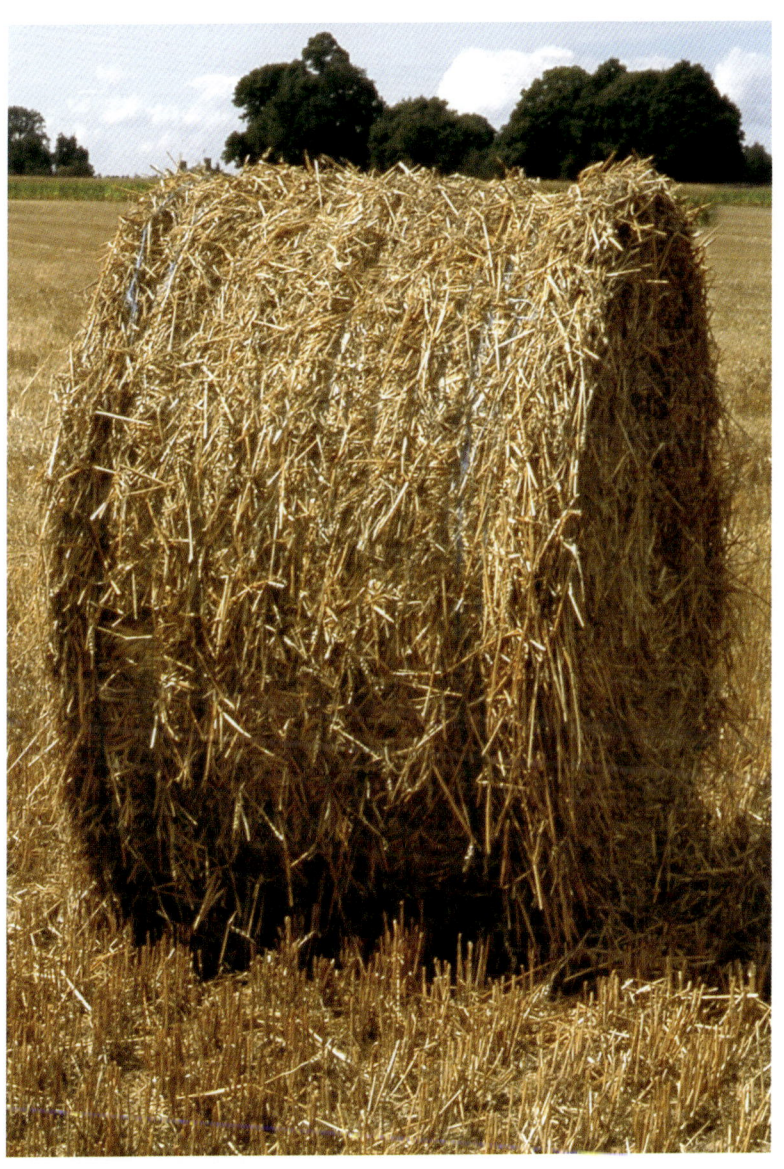

Take a moment to reflect:

Imagine an autumn season –

The rustle of the fallen leaves

The breeze catching the trees

The leaves crisp and dry

The autumn colours of burnished copper and gold

A chill in the air

There is a need to nurture

The nights are closing in

The smell of wood fires

A time of hibernation

The smell of roasting chestnuts.

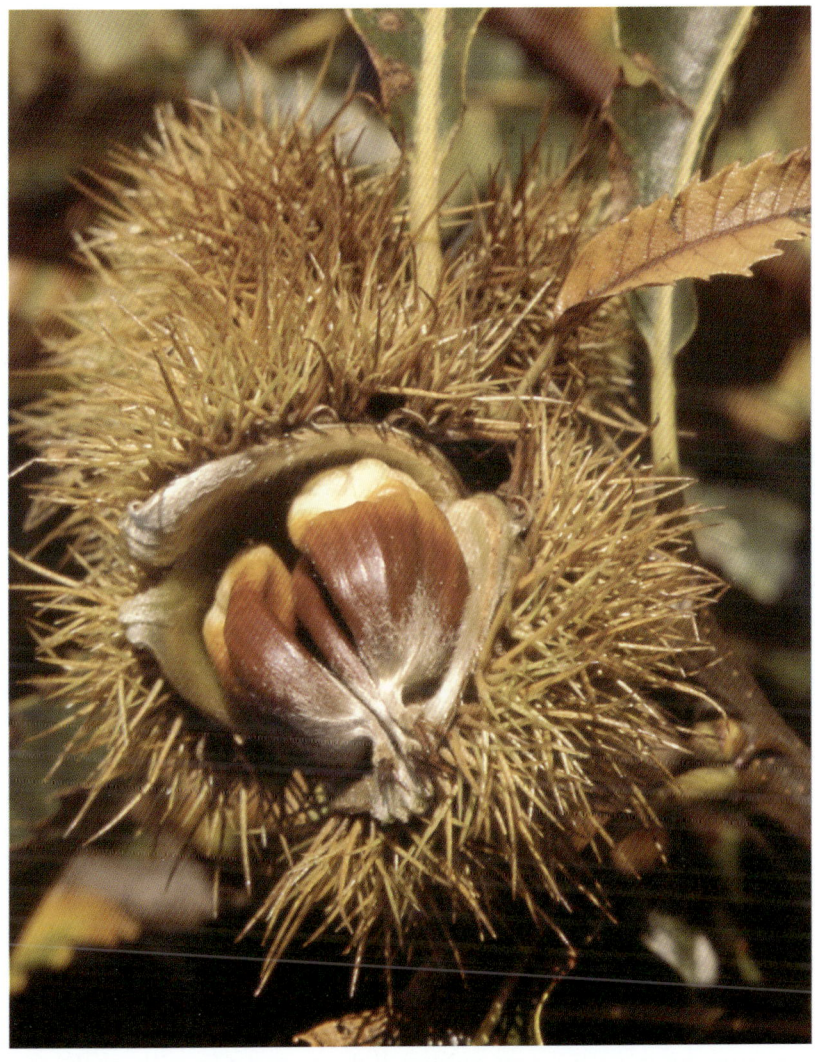

With every changing season there is wonder and beauty as nature begins her cycle once again. Transformation is change and within that comes balance.

Positive Imagery

Imagery is the mental representation of the human experience, which involves all your senses: sight, sound, touch, taste and smell. It can occur before, during or after external events, or in the absence of external events; for instance, when you dream. It represents a person's unique response to a situation. Imagery techniques help you to alter thoughts, feelings, attitudes and behaviour, which will then positively balance the mind's energy, to aid healing and recovery.

What you do, your actions and your behaviour, is preceded by an image of what will occur or what you may feel in any given situation. Your image of yourself and your life determines the way you relate to others and your environment. It may be that you feel a lack of self-confidence and this may ultimately increase your stress level, which will then have a direct effect on your immune system. Imagery can help to boost your immune system. Take a moment to think about the following:

- how do you perceive your cancer?

- how do you perceive radiotherapy, chemotherapy and surgery?

- how do you perceive your body?

Imagery can help you to focus positively on your cancer and on your treatment. It can also help to minimise the side effects of radiotherapy and chemotherapy. The following positive steps can help you to imagine your cancer and show you how imagery will help you fight it:

- go to a place that is comfortable and safe

- relax your body by concentrating on your breathing until you feel tranquil and peaceful

- now imagine a warm golden light moving in with each breath and all the tension leaving your body each time you breathe out.

When your body is relaxed, it's time to relax your mind. Choose one of the following images and focus your mind on it. Imagine:

- the face of someone you love

- eating your favourite food

- listening to your favourite music

- smelling your special perfume

- yourself on a beach

- your favourite room

- your favourite place

- you're a child again

Keep your mind focused. Let any thoughts drift in and out. Start by holding the image for one minute on the first day and slowly increase the time each day as you feel more confident using imagery. Remain relaxed with your body for a few minutes as you end the imagery.

Soul Moments

We all experience 'soul moments' in life – when we see a magnificent sunrise, hear the call of the loon, see the wrinkles in our mother's hands, or smell the sweetness of a bay. During these moments our body, as well as our brain, resonates as we experience the glory of being a human being.

Marion Woodman,
Taking Time To Just Be

Take a moment to reflect: can you list seven positive images? Use one each day of the week!

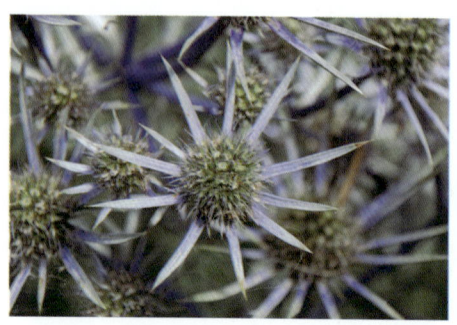

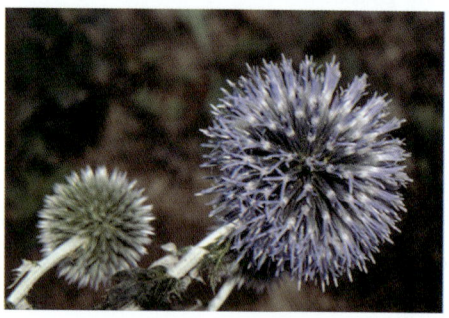

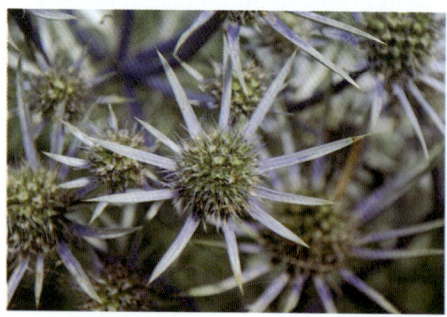

Nothing is as exhausting as indecision, and nothing more futile.

Bertrand Russell, *Begin It Now*

Living from the Inside Out: A Relationship with Yourself

Your ego invents endless reasons for you to remain upset with yourself. However, you can help release guilt and blame by replacing these emotions with forgiveness and love, once you have released your anger:

- vow never to repeat this or cause yourself pain again

- forgive yourself completely

Stubbornness is the language of the ego. You can dismantle barricades of past hurts by recognising the good in others and just accepting them as souls on their own journey. You may wish to remain stubborn and should therefore ask yourself why.

The relationship you have with yourself should positively support your self-esteem and confidence. Take a few moments to reflect on yours:

- what qualities do you have that cause you to love and respect yourself?

- list memories you have of feeling loved

- recall every friend you have ever made, every heart you have ever touched and every love you have ever shared

- write out the names and reflect upon each one in turn; remember them with affection

- write a poem or letter expressing your feelings towards someone who is a significant part of your life; let it come from your heart.

Your body language, the facial expressions and the intonation in your voice say much more about how you feel than words can ever say. Within a close, intimate relationship, a look or a touch conveys everything, without the need to say anything. You communicate at different levels every day, most of which are superficial, concerning the weather, what happened yesterday and what you are going to do today. But sometimes there is a need to communicate at a deeper level and this often makes you very vulnerable in that you may be giving out information that is very personal to you and at this level trust is essential.

This deeper level of communication is so vital when living with cancer and yet because you do not want to upset family and friends, it is a time when people are less able to say what they really mean, especially to those they love. It is important to remember that what you feel is often different from what you think. Thoughts trigger feelings, which then cause an emotional reaction which is often manifested in your behaviour.

The two steps that follow will help you to replace negative self-judgement of yourself with worthiness and loving kindness towards yourself. Use both steps each morning for as long as you need to. Write out this exact statement for each one of your negative qualities: I love and respect myself while taking positive steps to change. Tell someone you love what steps you are taking to replace your negative self-judgement.

Emotional well-being is about living fully in the moment, while looking and feeling great! Being 'sensory aware' is a measure of your capacity for life and is a gift to be cherished. You have the ability to recognise and express all aspects of your being: mind, body and spirit. The process of discovering your own unique truth will have special value and meaning if you are committed to 'doing it for yourself', rather than looking for someone else to 'do it for you'.

Cancer often allows you to evaluate your life and it can even give you a life-changing opportunity in that it may empower you to make changes. You may:

- surround yourself with people who can give you positive attention, care and unconditional love

- embark on a road to self-discovery and personal growth, in the face of adversity

- identify what is important in your life and let go of that which is no longer significant

- to be the best you can and to no longer seek perfection

- to be who you are and not what others think you should or would like you to be

- positively deal with the challenge of cancer and gain a new positive perspective

- love and respect yourself

- become non-judgemental

- set aside time for yourself, to do what is necessary to balance your mind, body and spirit

- be spontaneous, laugh and have fun

- reduce your stress, anxiety and tension levels

- explore complementary/expressive therapies

- decide to become who you are capable of being

- make each day count

- live each day as if it were your last

Giving yourself the opportunity to explore new ways of coping will help you to achieve harmony and balance in all areas of your life. It is about sustaining and maintaining you as a person in order to live life to the full, despite having cancer and the difficulties associated with treatment. You have the opportunity to be open and honest with yourself and those you love. You will always be a mother, daughter, employer, friend, brother, grandfather or father, but by giving yourself time, you can really explore who you are, without the need for a label. Self-healing comes from within. If you value your life and your survival, taking time to care for yourself is the most important thing you can do for yourself.

> Unconditional love knows no constraints.
> It is the most powerful healer of all.
> Love says: you matter
> Love says: you belong
> Love says: you make a difference.
>
> Daisy Goodwin, *101 Poems*

Take a moment to reflect: are you surrounded by people who give you positive attention, care and unconditional nurturing?

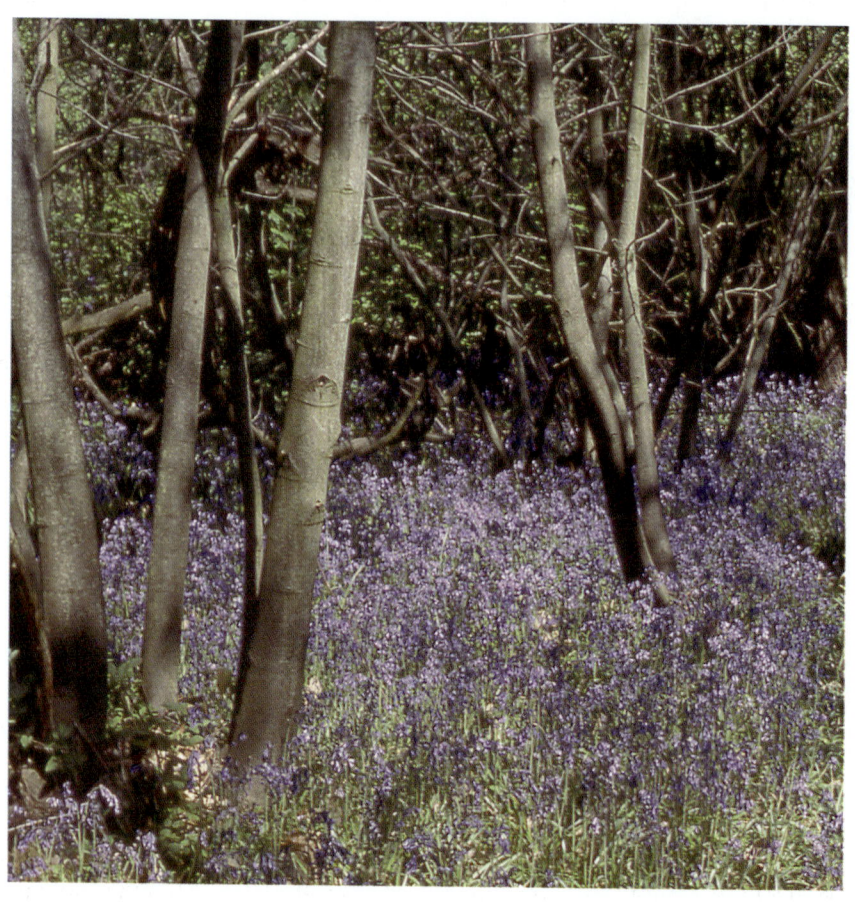

One of the great gifts of solitude is reflection and with reflection comes self-awareness.

Do You Say What You Mean? Do You Mean What You Say?

Your relationship with family and friends:
Often, words and language seem inadequate to try to explain what you are feeling to others. However, this is not a reason to stop trying. It is an opportunity to find other ways to express what you are feeling without the need for words.

To illustrate this, I recall an occasion when the consultant had just told someone's husband that he had lung cancer. Immediately, his wife stood up and accused her husband of being selfish. She told him he had brought this on himself because of the job he did, without a thought for his family. She then walked out of the consulting room. Words spoken in anger or fear are usually down to the thoughts and feelings of the angry individual. The issue for this gentleman's wife was her own fear of her husband not being there any more, together with guilt that she had been a smoker for many years.

If you want to try to understand what is going on in the mind of a person who has cancer remember, this is not about you or your relationship, it is about them and their cancer, so, do not:

- give advice

- say what you would do

- be defensive and dismissive

- take control of the situation

The only way you communicate back to them in this situation is through unconditional love. You cannot 'solve' the situation for them, but you can just hold them, hug them and be there for them. It is about 'being' not 'doing'.

One of the hardest things is to just listen to someone you love who is in so much emotional pain, as you will naturally want to take the pain away and make everything all right again. Sadly, you cannot take the pain away; you can only be there for them.

As in the example seen here, the wife had her own feelings to deal with, those of fear and guilt. Family and friends also need to recognise that they are also dealing with their own thoughts and feelings about cancer, which makes them feel insecure, frightened and sad. They also need to find support for themselves, someone to listen to them. The only way to get rid of feelings is to let them out, in a place that is safe for you.

Patient experience:

A young woman, Anne, had been through surgery for breast cancer and was about halfway through her chemotherapy. She had found a pattern emerging as she recovered from the treatment and she was becoming more and more angry with her family after each cycle of treatment. They would 'tiptoe' around her, saying nothing but acting as if everything was fine. When thinking about how she could get their attention to let them know what she was really going through, she decided to invite her family over for dinner one evening. She set the table in the kitchen, as the dining room was being redecorated at the time. After dinner everyone went through to the other room to see how the decorating was coming on.

As Anne went into the room she picked up an opened tin of cerise paint and threw it at the wall, to the horror of all who watched. Her husband had the foresight to ask why she had done that and she broke down, as did most of her family. She then tried to explain what living with cancer was like for her and how she wanted everyone to treat her as normal and not 'walk on eggshells' whilst they were around her. For the first time, they all sat down and really talked, honestly and openly.

At last, Anne could talk about her cancer and her treatment. It had taken something out of character for those around her to see what was really going on. Now, the dining room is finished, but it serves as a reminder of that day.

We expect people to know how we are feeling, but how can they when we do not tell them. We might say something like, 'How would you feel?', but how can they know how you feel? We presume they 'should know' or 'feel the same', but they don't! When discussing it with your family you need to:

- be clear about what is it that you want to say

- tell them what support you need from other people to help boost your fighting spirit

- think about the questions you want to ask and the possible answers you may get

- be aware that some of the reactions and answers you receive may be positive while others may be negative; can you deal with either response?

You will have ongoing concerns about your cancer and its treatment, and the impact it will have on your life. For you to remain in control, you need to learn to:

- communicate with yourself

- say what your feel

- communicate with others, making sure you always say what you mean

- be honest with yourself and others.

A Poem About Listening

When I ask you to listen to me and you start to give me advice, you have not done what I asked.

When I ask you to listen to me and you begin to tell me I shouldn't feel that way, you are trampling on my feelings.

When I ask you to listen to me and you feel you have to do something to solve my problems, you have failed me, strange as that may seem.

Listen! All I ask is that you listen to me, not talk or do – just hear me. Advice is cheap: 50p will get you both Claire Rayner and Russell Grant in the same newspaper.

And I can do for myself. I'm not helpless. Maybe discouraged and faltering, but not helpless. When you do something for me that I can and need to do for myself, you contribute to my fear and anxiety.

But when you accept as a simple fact that I do feel what I feel, no matter how irrational, then I can quit trying to convince you and get about the business of understanding what's behind this irrational feeling.

And when that's clear, the answers are obvious and I don't need advice. Irrational feelings make sense when we understand what's behind them.

So, please – listen and just hear me. And if you want to talk, wait a moment for your turn; and I'll listen to you.

Anon

Take a moment to reflect: do you say what you mean? Do you mean what you say?

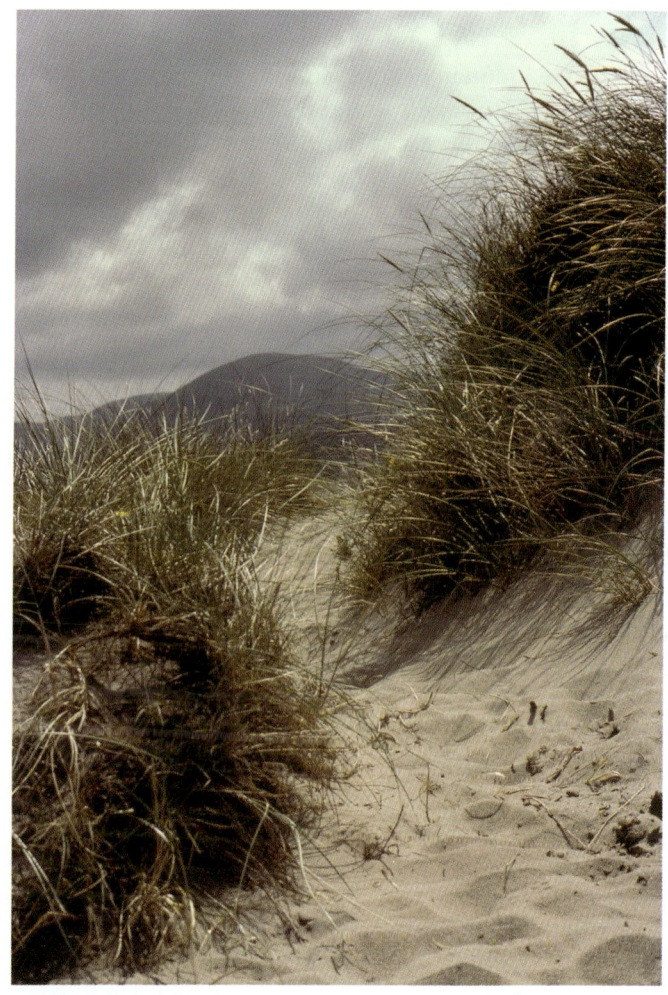

Love who you are and what you are and what you do. Laugh at yourself and at life and nothing can touch you. It's all temporary anyway. Next lifetime you will do it differently, so why not do it differently now?

Louise Hay, *Bag of Jewels*

Art and Music Expression

> Music is the poetry of sound.
>
> Jim Billingsley, *Reflections*

When words are inadequate, expression through art or music may help. The use of colour, texture and sound may help you to explore what you are thinking or feeling at any given moment. Children learn to draw instinctively and spontaneously from a very early age and their art reflects their moods and feelings. Art is now widely used in hospitals and schools. Art and music expression is about transferring onto paper what you think and feel and then letting it go!

Within this section I shall relate several patients' experiences of using art and music. In the appendix you can find templates on how you can explore art and music therapy for yourself.

Patient experience – the inside/out box:

Graham struggled to find himself and so I gave him a pile of magazines and a shoebox and asked him if he could use the pictures and words in the magazine to decorate the outside of the box with images that he was happy to portray to other people about himself.

I then asked him to put inside the box pictures of who he really was, maybe a side that he does not want others to see or perhaps a side of him that he could not bear to look at. About an hour later he asked to see me.

He showed me the outside of the box, which had pictures of him as a husband, father, brother and son, pictures of who he represented in his job, the car he drove and the sports he played and he talked me through all those roles he played each day.

He then opened the box, and I was surprised to see that all that was inside was a black piece of paper. He looked at me and said he was so busy being all the things on the outside of the box that he didn't know who he really was any more.

He went on to say that he was not the person on the outside of the box; however, people saw him always in a role. Since his cancer was diagnosed, he felt he had let everyone down, as he could no longer carry out all those roles. Unable to let anyone know how he was feeling or how to express his fears, inside he felt empty, alone and forgotten.

Over the next few weeks he began to explore who he was inside the box and in so doing he began to learn about his true self. He had to confront what cancer meant to him and how he would learn to deal with that. He also learnt new ways of getting through the chemotherapy.

His cancer journey took several months and about a year after I had seen the black inside 'the box', he showed me who he had now become. His life now had meaning since he had confronted his fear of cancer. It had been a positive life-changing experience both for him and for all his friends and family. He has always kept that shoebox, as it serves as a powerful reminder of his need to find himself and be true to himself.

Patient experience – do not presume:

A patient once told me of a Christmas present that she dreaded getting every year from her husband. Her husband knew how house-proud she was and how she liked the home to be clean and tidy, so each year he gave her something to help her clean the house, such as a vacuum cleaner! Each year she said it was lovely and looked surprised, but she never actually told her husband how she really felt. Instead, each year she hoped he would give her a new dress, perfume or jewellery.

Now, having expressed her feelings, he knows just how she felt and she is full of hope that this year's Christmas present will be special. We should never presume other people know how you are feeling. They don't. They need you to tell them.

Take a moment to reflect: what would the outside and inside of your shoebox look like?

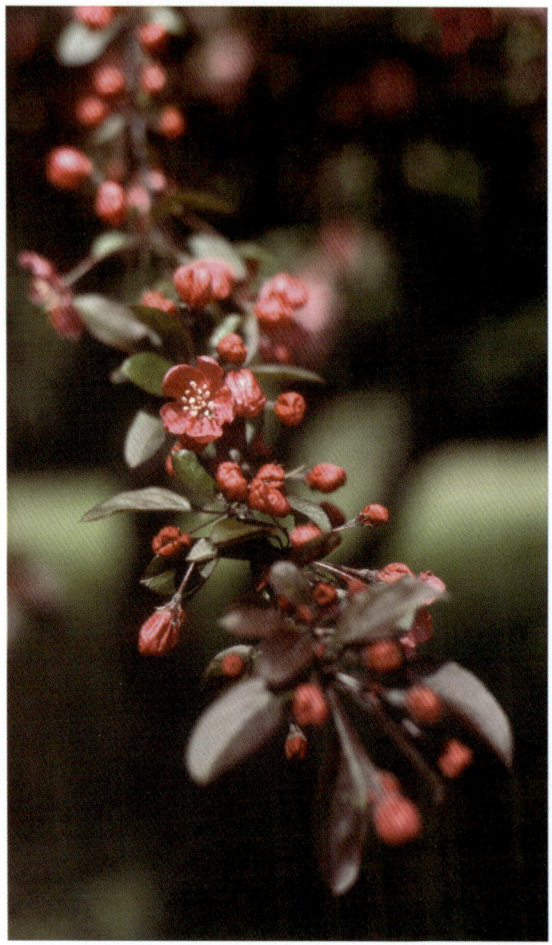

What is right for one soul may not be right for another. It may mean having to stand on your own and do something strange in the eyes of others. But do not be daunted. Do whatever it is because you know within it is right for you.

Eileen Caddy, *Bag of Jewels*

Patient experience – in the picture:

One patient told me that she had used the 'in the picture' illustration on two occasions. The first one was two months after being diagnosed with cancer and what she found was that she appeared in the centre of the picture, but all her family and friends were on the edges of the paper, The only person close to her on the picture was her oncologist. The picture helped her to realise that in her attempt to protect those she loved and cared for, she was pushing them away. At that time the oncologist held her life in his hands. He had control of her life and she did not know how to get her life back. When she talked it through with her family and friends they had no idea what she was feeling. Several months later I met her again and she pulled out of her handbag a picture she had recently done. She still remained in the centre, but the rest of the picture was full of people. I asked her to show me the oncologist and there at the edge of the paper was a doctor running out! When you look at the power of positive images, it is evident to see how you can change negative thoughts into positive ones.

Patient experience – create your own story:

That is exactly what another patient did whilst waiting each day in the radiotherapy department for her treatment. Each day, she took a picture with her that had caught her eye in a magazine. She would sit in the waiting room and take out the picture and then create a story in her journal of what was happening in that picture:

- immediately before the picture was taken

- in the picture now

- after the picture was taken

- If you were using this method of expression, would you be in the story either before, now or in the future?

- The ability to learn new ways to perceive and interpret life's challenges is the greatest gift of being human. You can choose to make a real difference in your own recovery. Sharing this with others allows everyone to understand what is going on for you!

Take a moment to reflect: are you hanging on to the past? If so, ask yourself why. Yesterday was just a dream, tomorrow a vision of hope, but today is for living.

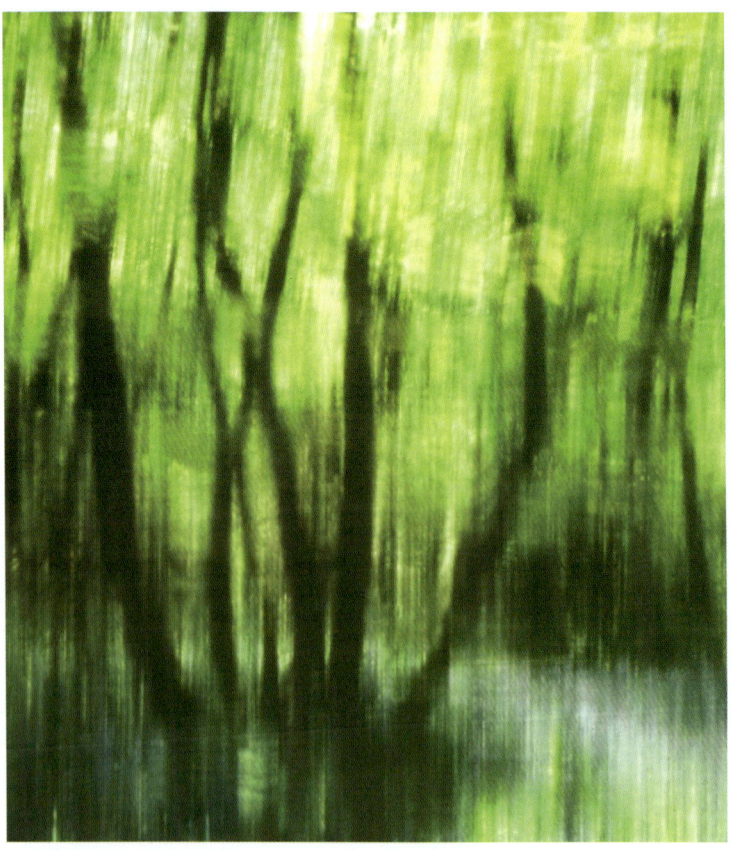

Music allows you a different medium of expression and the healing power of music has been recognised for centuries. In Western society, the true benefits of music have begun to come into their own as a form of therapy. Psychiatrists discovered that the power of music helped patients to relax and release pent-up emotions. Obstetricians have used the pulsating sounds of music in Special Care Baby Units (SCBU) to help infants develop their fighting spirit. The use of music to heal, relax and promote wellness is now used in many different medical situations. Music is both powerful and emotive and it can evoke different moods and feelings. Music can:

- increase vitality or induce relaxation

- be used as a specific theme for socialisation

- enhance well-being if used in conjunction with therapeutic touch, such as massage or reiki

Music is intimately personal; music to one person's ears can be pain to another's. This is part of what makes us uniquely individual. Talking about your music preference can not only release emotion but also aid communication with others.

Music to move to:

Try playing one of your favourite CDs. Turn the volume up loud and move with the music. Sing the words and let the rhythm take hold of you and move with it. What do you feel? Anger, sadness, elation, comforted, empowered? What memories came flooding back? Use your journal to express them.

Patient experience – fighting spirit music:

One patient played a very expressive cd in her car on the way to her hospital appointments. It reminded her of rallying the troops and marching forward, to win her personal battle against cancer.

After all her chemotherapy finished, she found that she could not listen to that cd again. It had served its purpose at the time, but that was now behind her. Other patients have found that using relaxing music whilst having chemotherapy helps them through the treatment.

Patient experience – engage with life:

I found that much of the time I was surrounded by silence and therefore had a lot of time to think, which was not always helpful. Our home was never quiet and so it was alien to me when suddenly my son stopped playing his music in his room. Why was this? I knew my son would give me the most honest reply, so I asked him outright. What he said was that nothing felt right any more. No one knew what to say or do and so we all just moved around the house ignoring each other.

It made me realise that sometimes you need to tell the family that it's all right for things to be normal. He gave me a hug and then went straight upstairs and pumped up the music volume. We both sighed with relief!

Mood music:

On a wet afternoon, why not put on a cd and close your eyes, relax and let the music wash over you. Recall how you felt: before you put the music on, while it was playing and after the music stopped. Did the music invigorate you or relax you? Instead of writing what you feel, it may help to paint or draw the feelings that came to mind. Where did the music take you?

Patient experience – music to play and heal:

A young guy found his chemotherapy difficult, especially as he was also in isolation. His friends clubbed together and invested in an iPod for him and downloaded all his favourite music onto it. He was delighted by the gift and before each of his treatment cycles he plugged in his music and relaxed during each treatment. After seven days he changed his music to hard rock, knowing that his immune system needed to recover within the next ten days in order for him to be well enough for his next cycle of treatment and to take him on the way to recovery. It got him through a difficult time and he felt that he was able in some way to control his fight back from cancer.

Many patients find music excellent for relaxation purposes, but it is important that you find the right music for you to relax to. Listen to the cd to make sure the voice, the accent, the orchestration and the lyrics are right for you. The wrong music can cause you stress! Music can be used to motivate or to relax, or even just to enjoy!

Take a moment to reflect: what music uplifts you, relaxes you or encourages your fighting spirit? What music lets you show or release those emotions when you are on your own? Maybe the beauty of today is music!

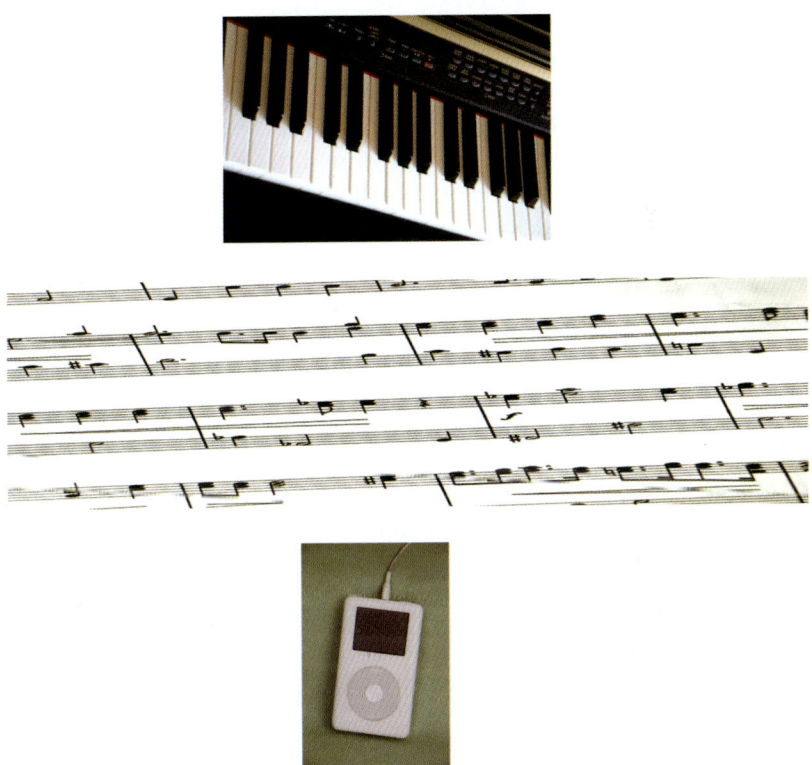

.... there is a real danger of overlooking a very important day ... today. For this is the place and the time for living. Let us live each day abundantly and beautifully while it is here.

Esther Baldwin York, *Taking Time To Just Be*

Mind Methods of Healing

Facing cancer is stressful. This may manifest as a strong emotional response which may make you feel:

- out of control, or

- that you will lose control

It is essential that your sense of personal control over the cancer is not lost or taken over by the professionals who are treating your cancer or by members of your family. It is important that you decide the best course of treatment for you and commit to that, in order for you to regain control over the cancer and your life. The essence of who you are will facilitate your personal pathway to self-healing and make your recovery worth fighting for and your life worth living. Taking responsibility for your own recovery will allow you to reduce stress and replace it with an auspicious healing environment that is filled with peace and love.

Do you see the glass half full or half empty? How you view the glass identifies if you think from a positive or a negative place. You can use positive affirmations to change your mindset. Positive affirmations facilitate positive goal-setting. Goal-setting means that your life has meaning and purpose, however, you should not have to pursue them either through effort and struggle. Be aware that when setting goals, you may feel resistance. Think about why that might be, what is causing it and whether it will ultimately prevent you from achieving your goal.

Remember:

- keep your goals simple and realistic

- choose goals that you can achieve and accomplish

- phrase them in a direct, upbeat way

- when you achieve your goal, congratulate and reward yourself

- set short-term goals, once an hour, once a day, once a week or once a month, as well as long-term goals

- don't try to achieve all your goals at once

- embracing the true concept of your inner healer means acknowledging its work at every level in mind, body and spirit.

- self-healing comes from within!

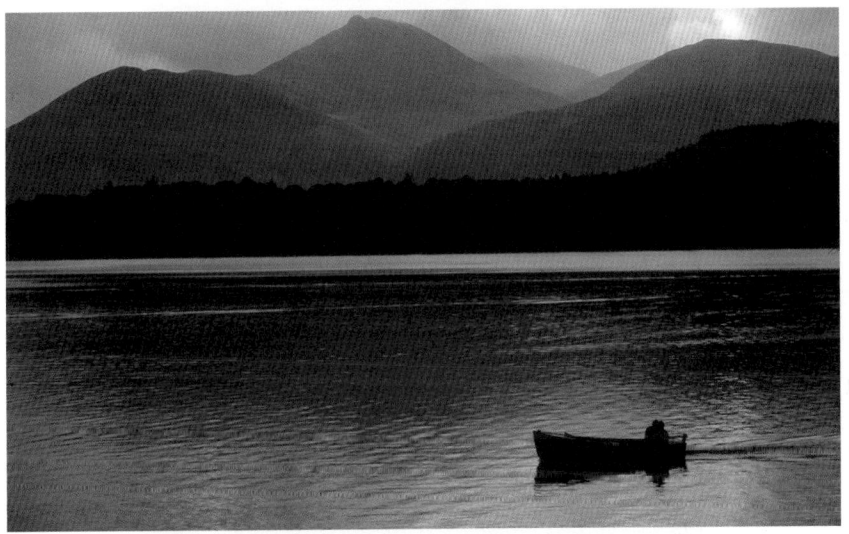

A shaft of sunlight at the end of a dark afternoon, a note in music, and the way the back of a baby's neck smells ... These are the really important things.

E. B. White, *Taking Time To Just Be*

Take a moment to reflect: what life-enhancing goals can you set yourself for the next three months?

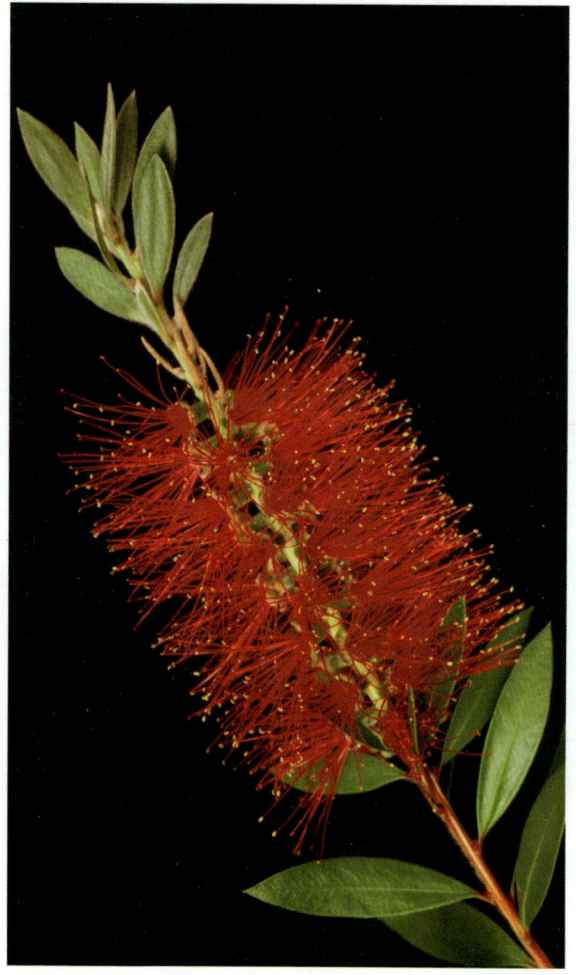

We achieve a sense of self from what we do ourselves and how we develop our capabilities. If all your efforts have gone into developing others, you're bound to feel empty. Take your turn now!

Robin Norwood, *Bag of Jewels*

Talking Therapies

As our bodies struggle to maintain health and well-being, so do our minds. The mind–body connection demonstrates that you need to treat the mind and body together. Complementary therapies help to relax and heal the body and restore its balance, whereas psychological therapies aim to relax and heal the mind and restore its balance. It is about addressing thoughts and emotions that are difficult to deal with on your own. Working with a therapist or a counsellor can allow you to talk things through that may otherwise be difficult to discuss with those closest to you. There are many types of therapy and here are just a few:

Cognitive behavioural therapy:

This works on the premise that thoughts of low self-worth are incorrect and are as a result of faulty learning. The aim of therapy is to get rid of faulty concepts that influence negative thinking.

Analytical psychology:

This type of therapy regards a person's mindset as the outcome of conflict between internal forces and it seeks answers from the unconscious. It aims to uncover and analyse the effects of early experiences on present difficulties and to look at ways of working to resolve early blocks.

Humanistic psychology:

This optimistic view emphasises the essential goodness of human beings and the belief that we all have choices. In order to realise your full potential, you need to get in touch with your inner self, acknowledge your feelings and find new ways of expressing them. The therapist and client work from a position of equality.

Integrative psychology:

Most therapists who work in this way have a humanistic orientation but also use elements of other therapeutic disciplines, such as psychosynthesis, Gestalt and transpersonal or existential psychotherapy. Its ruling principle is the integration of mind, body and soul to constitute one whole, aware individual.

Hypnotherapy:

Healing a patient who is in a state of trance is one of the oldest therapeutic arts. Many scientists have struggled to explain hypnotherapy and how it works. It is one of the few therapies taught in medical schools and is considered to be a useful method of encouraging healing by altering behavioural states. In the hands of a qualified practitioner, hypnotherapy is completely safe. Self-hypnosis is also safe and most health conditions may find benefit from using this practice. Hypnotherapy can draw upon all the vast resources of the unconscious mind, which is why it can be so effective in helping a wide range of problems and addictions.

These are just a few of the therapies available these days and I suggest that if you want to explore them, you should find a qualified practitioner, especially someone with knowledge of cancer and its treatment. Meet the therapist to see what they have to offer and to see if you feel comfortable and can relate to them.

Most cancer centres now provide or have access to a counsellor, a psychotherapist or a cognitive behavioural therapist. If your hospital, GP or clinic is unable to provide this service, then contact BACUP, Macmillan Cancer Relief, Breast Cancer Care or the British Association of Counselling and Psychotherapy for a list of therapists in your area.

Meditation, imagery and relaxation form part of the work you have to do in order to rebalance your energy. But to treat you and help you on your way towards relaxation, you should make an appointment to see an aromatherapist, a reflexologist or a reiki therapist, letting someone else do the work.

Take a moment to reflect: who do you feel that you can really talk to?

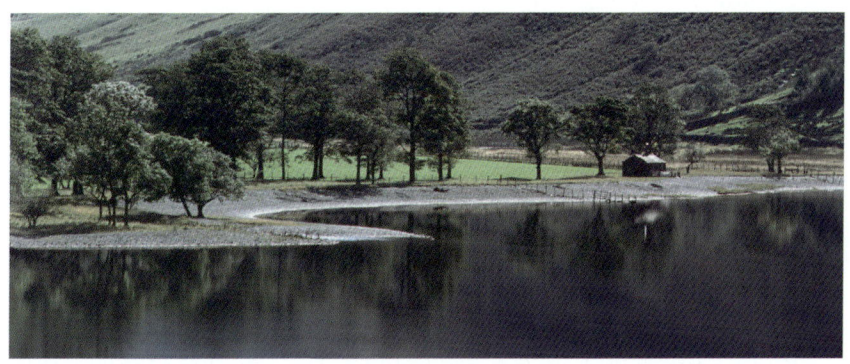

Even in the heart of the city there can be a place of calm. Doors shut and curtains closed, a light against the dark, wrapped around dear accustomed things we can withdraw and find ourselves again.

Pam Brown, *Taking Time To Just Be*

Laughter Therapy

What comes from the heart touches the heart.

Don Sibet, *Bag of Jewels*

Can you find the joy in living and laughing?

- Can you remember the last time you were really excited? What did it feel like?

- Did you feel happy, carefree, like nothing bothered you?

- Do you need some excitement in your life?

- When did you last feel special?

- Can you remember the excitement of Christmas?

- Can you remember the fun of birthdays, or walking in the rain, or of being in love?

- Has your cancer taken these feelings away? Well, you have the power to control your thoughts and feelings.

- Can you see the funny side of things?

- Can you laugh at yourself?

If you cannot sleep, then listen to a tape of your favourite comedy, or take time to think of silly things you did and instead of reprimanding yourself, laugh at it. When you wake, take a few moments to think about the things you are looking forward to today. Do something for you each day and put some fun back in your life. Read that book you have always wanted to; buy yourself some special bath oil or a bunch of flowers. Take time out to watch a programme or a DVD. Enjoy a massage or a manicure as you continue your journey to wellness.

Just before you go to sleep, think back over the day and recall things that you were grateful for, like an unexpected phone call or a friend visiting. Think of the things that really made you laugh and feel alive.

Would you say it is a joy to be alive? If not, how can you make it so? Cancer is serious, but your life does not have to be so serious. Where is your spontaneity?

- go out and buy yourself or better still make yourself a thank-you card for all you have achieved.

- for all you have shared and experienced in life and for all those who you love up to this point, send them a funny card and watch their reaction

- but don't stop there, make yourself a best wishes card for the future or good luck card, for all the beauty, love and joy that is still to come in your life

■ start a laughter group and arrange for you and your friends to meet for coffee once a week, to share jokes, events and comical books or to watch a humorous DVD. Everyone will have a specific type of humour that they like, so get to know other people by finding out what makes them laugh!

Take a moment to reflect: give yourself the gift of unconditional love, inner strength, laughter and fun and informed choice.

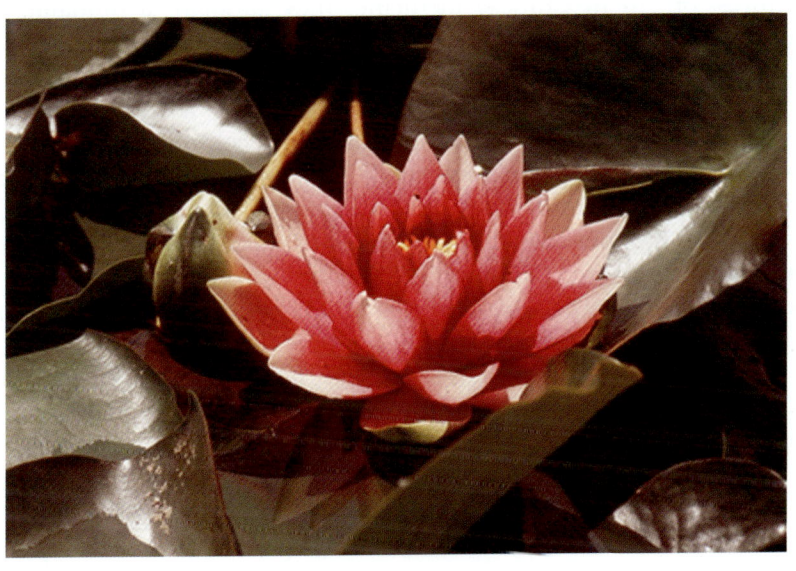

Life's a pretty precious and wonderful thing:
You can't sit down and let it lap around you ...
You have to plunge into it; you have to dive through it.

Kyle Crichton, *Bag of Jewels*

Mind–Body Connection

Psychobiology is the name of the science that gives us new understanding of how exactly the mind and body communicate and how this can help you to promote your own self-healing. Thoughts, feelings and emotions influence not only our health but also the appearance and cause of physical and psychological disease. With every thought there is a chemical reaction, which alters your mind and body's energy balance.

Almost all traditions of medicine, apart from Western medicine, are based on the concept of life energy. Whether prana, as in Indian cultures, or chi in Chinese medicine, they all share a fundamental understanding of energy as the vital force that flows through every living thing. To achieve holistic health and maintain it is to arrive at a point of balance where the energies of the mind, body and spirit are one! You can choose to either assist nature in accomplishing its healing work by supporting your mind, body and spirit energies or you can choose a descent into illness and disease by subjecting yourself to addictive habits, negative thought processes and a lack of meaning and purpose in your life. The mind has the ability to be either slayer or a healer. In other words, what is in your mind and in your heart can make you sick or well accordingly.

By being actively engaged in your own health and life choices, you do not become totally dependent on: a doctor, a hospital, surgical procedures and medication. Toxic emotions such as unresolved conflict, fear, anger, loneliness and despair send your body a 'give up' message or increase negative energy, while forgiveness, love, kindness and hope become transformed into a powerful communication between cells that invites peace of mind and sends positive messages of healing and life.

The mind is the vehicle within each human organism that regulates and controls all of its systems, be it metabolic, nervous, circulatory or hormonal. Treating cancer does not mean the rest of your life has to fit around it, rather the reverse – the treatment has to fit around your life.

Patient experience:

I needed to have fifteen radiotherapy treatments at my regional cancer centre for my breast cancer. I decided to wear a special and different outfit each day that I attended. It helped me to be proud of who I was and to feel good about myself and my new body image. It was a way of saying look at me, I am here and I will beat this cancer.

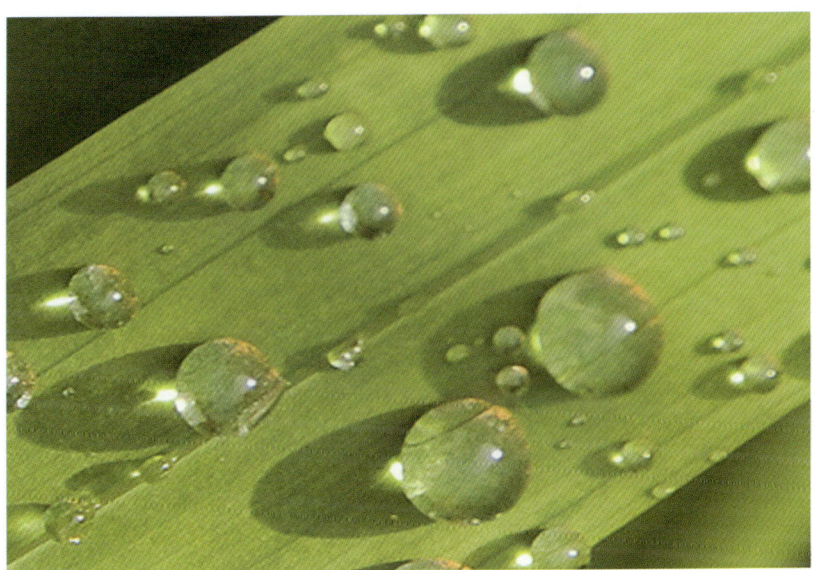

Take a moment to reflect: take this opportunity to identify what is important in your life and let go of what is not.

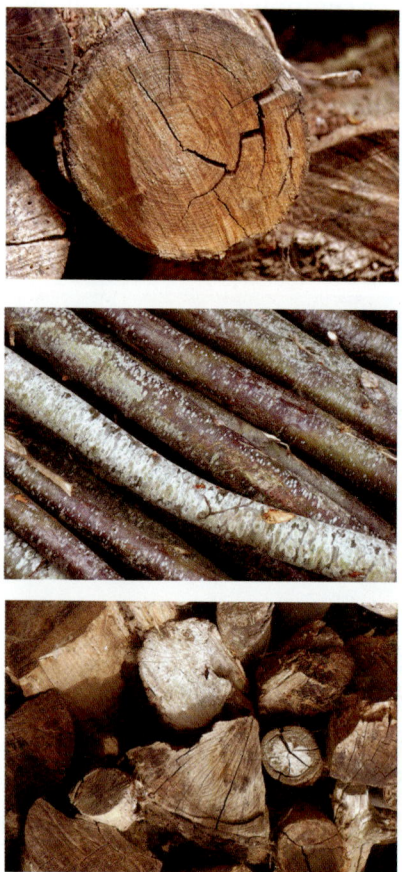

Suppose you went at a slow pace …
To feel your body, play with children,
Look openly without agenda or timetable
Into the faces of those you loved.
Suppose you took time each day to sit in silence,
I think if you did these things, the world wouldn't need much saving.

Donella H. Meadows, *Taking Time To Just Be*

Cancer and the Body

Body Wellness

When diagnosed with cancer, no doubt one of the first things you asked was what caused my cancer. There is no simple answer to this complex question, because the causes are many and varied. There are more than a hundred different cancers, all of which have different triggers, many of which are still unknown.

To achieve body wellness, firstly you need to assess what is causing any imbalance of your body's energy. The following five main factors will be covered in more depth later in this section.

- nutrition

- exercise

- hygiene and safety

- de-addiction

- stress

Achieving optimum health is a lifetime goal. Wellness is much more than the absence of disease. Ultimately, your health depends more on what you are willing to do for yourself, rather than what others are willing to do for you. Initially, as you go through surgery, radiotherapy or chemotherapy, it will take all your energy and determination to heal the body both during and after treatment. The treatment goes on for several weeks or months and during this period it allows you time for reflection. It may be that you wish to reflect on your lifestyle or refocus on the important things in your life. Or you may wish to reduce the risk of being diagnosed with another or a secondary cancer, by changing your diet or environment. The journey towards wellness is just as important as the goal, so you should embrace activities that inspire you and make you feel good about yourself.

Self-replicating DNA transmits the genetic information of every individual, passing it from one generation to another. Our internal biological clock highlights when our body is changing, through the effects that hormones have on the body during adolescence, adulthood and old age. The templates of the diseases that are carried in our genetic make-up are usually locked within our cells forever, a few of which are never meant to appear, but those that do resurface must wait for the correct signals from your body.

Certain types of disease tend naturally to appear at certain stages of life or when your energy is out of balance, maybe because of your lifestyle, such as eating processed foods, inactivity, anxiety, fear, addictions, environmental changes and pollution. All of these triggers cause damage to your cells and create an imbalance day by day and week by week.

There are over 100 different types of cancer and it has been estimated that 80 per cent of these are environmentally influenced. The effects of stress also have a devastating effect on your immune system and its ability to recognise and eliminate malignant cells.

Cancer is a complex process, involving some factors that you can control, as well as some factors that you cannot. The foods we eat, the toxins we knowingly ingest, the ways we use our five senses and how we express our emotions are all under our control.

When you consider the human body as more than the sum of its various parts and recognise it as a collection of cells vibrating with energy, then rather than being constrained by information, we can expand our wisdom and begin regarding our bodies in a new light, as energy. In the body, discord and 'dis-ease' occurs when the energy of your cells is out of balance. Western medicine uses a diagnosis such as asthma, diabetes and cancer for identifying disease. It also enhances and prolongs life by relieving symptoms of illness and by removing diseased parts of the body. But what it does not do is help to heal the mind and spirit.

> The grand essentials to happiness in this life are something to do, something to love, and something to hope for.
>
> Joseph Addison, *Bag of Jewels*

Take a moment to reflect: can you think of a reason why your body's energy is out of balance?

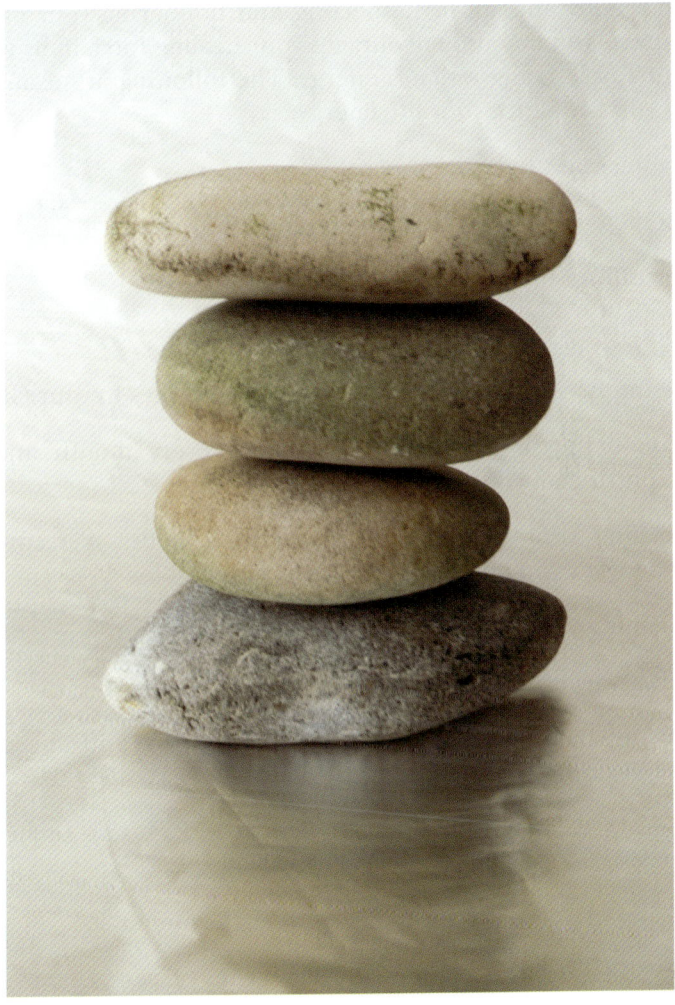

Life was never meant to be a struggle; just a gentle progression from one point to another, much like walking through a valley on a sunny day.

Stuart Wilde, *Bag of Jewels*

Your Body's Energy System

Wellness is the dance of life that celebrates infinite harmony between the mind, body and spirit. Respecting and honouring your body not only protects you but also encourages your healing force in its work, so that your whole being radiates energy. The following are examples of activities that enhance your life energy:

- being safe rather than sorry

- being outside enjoying nature whenever possible

- brushing your teeth at least twice a day

- practising safe sex

- being Breast Aware and reporting any changes to your GP

- conducting a testicular examination every month and reporting any changes to your GP

- locking your doors and ensuring the house is secure whenever you leave it, as well as at night

- keeping your body clean and in good condition

- always using a seat belt in a car

- using sunscreen and avoiding prolonged and direct exposure to intense sunlight

- having regular smear test (female) or PSA test (male) (prostate screening)

- living in a smoke-free home/work environment

- avoiding dark and potentially dangerous places

- engaging in a healthy, loving, committed relationship

- looking for natural alternatives to work in parallel with Western medicines

- finding the root cause of the problem rather than just treating the symptoms

Taking responsibility for your health and caring for your body is a lifetime commitment. Only by constantly assessing your body's wellness, and changing your lifestyle accordingly, can you hope to remain in optimum health.

Whilst receiving chemotherapy or radiotherapy it is important to listen to what your body is telling you and respond accordingly to maintain wellness. The treatment for cancer not only kills the cancer cells but also healthy cells as well and your immune system may therefore be unable to fight off an infection. If you are feeling unwell, give your oncology department a ring – it will reduce your anxiety but you also receive advice on what you need to do if the symptoms persist.

Many patients, both during and following treatment, have experienced symptoms such as a sore throat or flu and they immediately think the cancer has returned or spread. Often this is not the case, a sore throat is just a sore throat and feeling lethargic may be flu or simply that you have done too much. But it is always advisable to check it out with your oncologist or specialist nurse.

To achieve wellness is to obtain the point of balance where the energies of mind, body and spirit are finely attuned to each other, so that the distinctions between them fade away.

The Body's Rhythm for Life

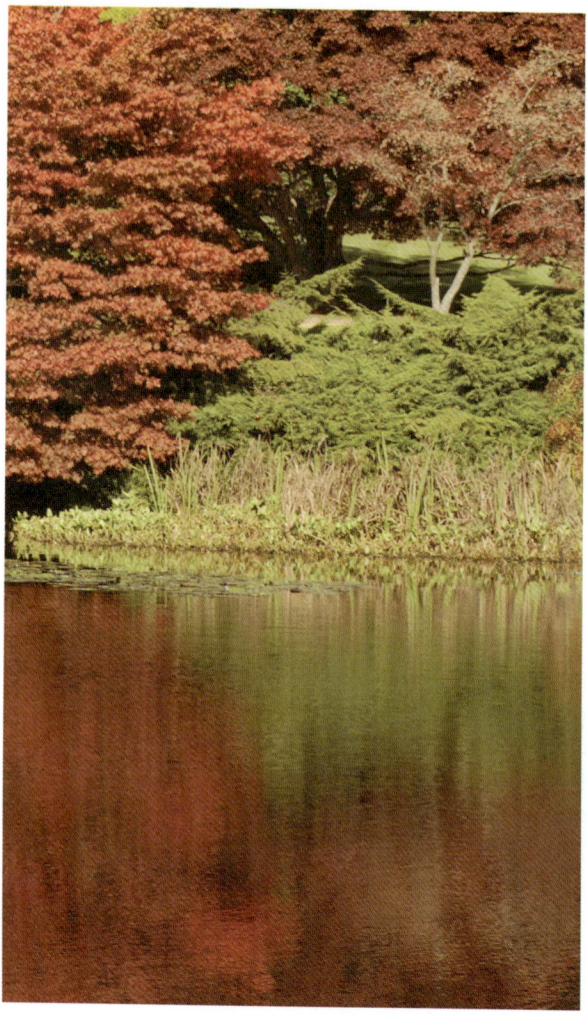

Take a moment to reflect: how was your body's energy before you were diagnosed with cancer? What do you need to do to achieve body wellness?

Life is an opportunity and not an obligation.

The Toa of Leadership, *Bag of Jewels*

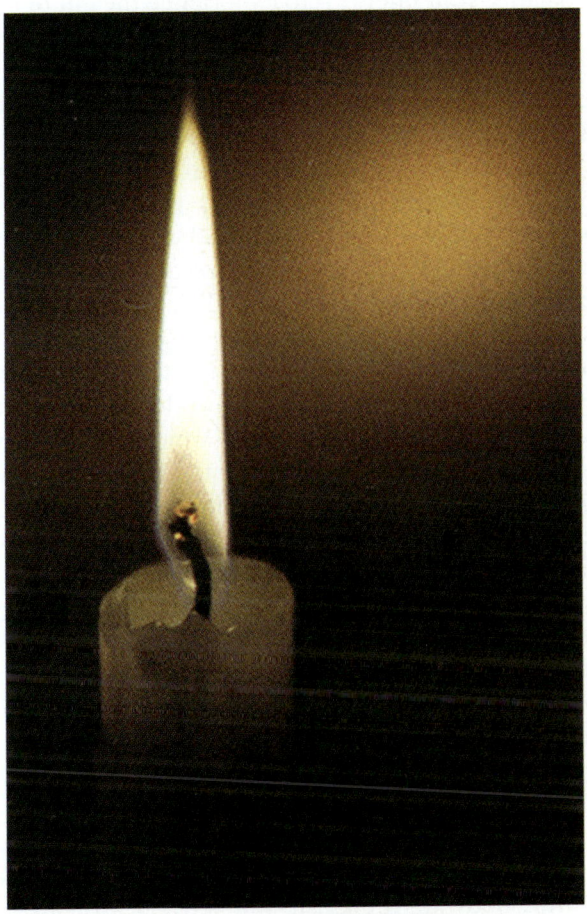

We learn wisdom from failure much more than from success. We often discover what will do, by finding out what will not do; and probably he who never made a mistake never made a discovery.

Samuel Smiles, *Begin It Now*

Your Body Energy Balanced

If we perceive illness and disease as energy out of balance, we have the ability to actively restore the energy flow within our mind, body and spirit. To rebalance your energy is to experience the gift of life as a state of vibrant, radiant wellness.

Human beings are not programmed to self-destruct. Our genes are intended to enable the preservation, protection and survival of our species. This intention exists deep within the heart of every individual as 'remembered wellness'. Your infinite wisdom maintains your inner compass that is always pulled towards wellness.

Remembered wellness exists even behind veils of illness and disease. It continually attempts to create harmony, restore balance and maintain life. This truth remains, however ill the body may be, it is always possible to experience a breakthrough to wellness.

The most effective health care seeks to treat the whole person. Many older traditions of healing, combining the understanding of the human ensemble, are seen as a threefold entity which intrinsically links the mind, body and spirit and strives to restore the health of the whole body. These therapies are known as complementary therapies or energy therapies and are carried out by qualified and registered practitioners.

Every illness is anchored on an imbalance of energy. The real choice we have is not to become dependent on doctors, hospitals, surgery procedures and medication, but to learn to mobilise our own healing force, awakening its spirit, to achieve a balance of energy. The following five factors can be under your control, to help maintain your energy balance:

Nutrition:

This is about eating healthy and wholesome food that nourishes the mind, body and spirit. A nurturing diet is one that is balanced and encourages the body to replenish vital energy instead of draining energy in the process of digestion.

Exercise:

This is about finding an energetic activity you enjoy two to three times a week, for a period of thirty minutes. It will also strengthen your body and calm your mind. Exercise revitalises your body's storehouse of energy, to stimulate your healing force.

Hygiene and safety:

This is about investing time to care for your body. Respecting and honouring your body protects and encourages your healing force, so that your whole being radiates life energy.

De-addiction:

This is about releasing yourself from substances and habits that harm your mind, body and spirit. It helps to build your self-esteem and self-worth. It reminds you of the reverence for life and cares for the soul, so that harmful habits melt away.

Stress:

This is about acknowledging that your body needs to reduce your levels of stress. It is about recognising that you need to sleep, to allow the body to repair and heal itself. Allowing time for rest and relaxation during the day is essential, especially during and after receiving surgery, chemotherapy or radiotherapy or after an illness.

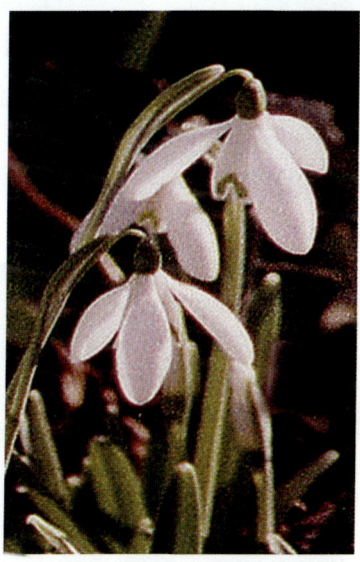

Nothing can bring you peace but yourself.

Ralph Waldo Emerson, *Begin It Now*

Take a moment to reflect: assessing your body energy now, is it balanced or unbalanced? Have your body's energy levels changed?

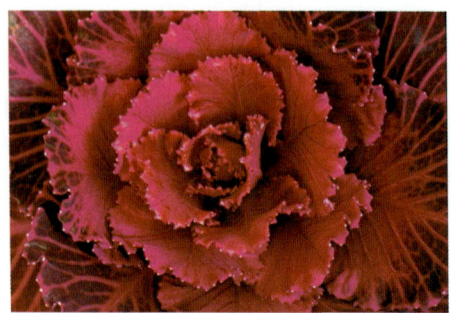

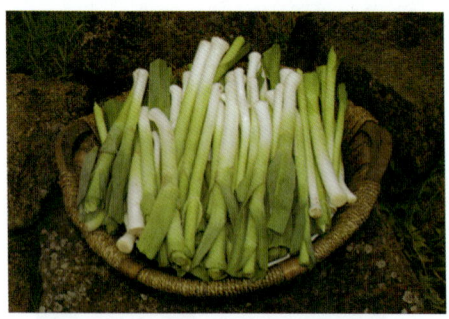

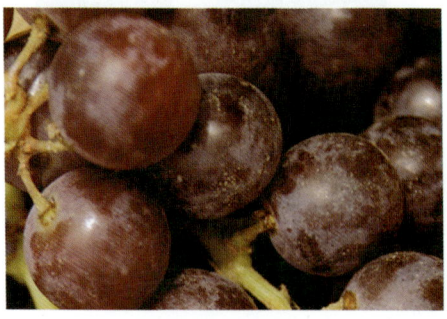

Procrastination is the thief of time.

Edward Young, *Begin It Now*

Your Body Energy Unbalanced

You may experience or feel many of the following signs and symptoms that indicate a disturbed energy balance:

- the universe is basically unfriendly and your life is out of control

- enslaved by; alcohol, tobacco or drugs

- prolonged periods of gloom and despondency where you rarely see lightness in life

- cause yourself and others deliberate hurt

- difficulty controlling bad habits and allowing stress to overcome your resolve

- weight problems, exercise infrequently and prefer to avoid challenges

- a general dissatisfaction with life and lacking a clear purpose, plan or intent

- seek quick fixes for difficulties and rarely try to discover the root cause of a problem

- your energy flow is impeded

- your natural healing force has become suppressed, but is striving to restore energy balance

Fortunately, your potential to be well is great. You have sufficiently high regard for life to want to look and feel good. Greater effort to care for your mind, body and spirit will empower you to develop higher levels of balanced energy that will enhance your potential for complete wellness.

Remember that ill health indicates lack of love in your life. The key to restoring the energy balance is forgiveness and love for yourself and others. Nourishing yourself with kindness and compassion reaps dramatic health rewards. The ultimate responsibility for positively caring for your body is up to you. While you have been struggling to maintain your energy balance, your natural healing force has been overcome. Your energy flow is blocked and if not rectified, energy disharmony eventually becomes disease.

Do not despair and never give in, as even the smallest effort to revive your healing force can begin to restore your body's harmony and balance. It is never too late to take the very first step towards better self-care. If, however, your lifestyle and the choices you make are not supporting your health, then you will be pursuing a path that will just hasten your body's natural decline and accelerate the appearance of disease. Your health and happiness requires a substantial commitment and ongoing concentrated effort. You can build strength and enhance your attitude by taking steps to change at least some of your self-destructive habits.

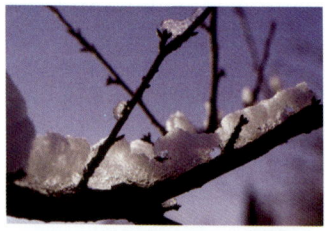

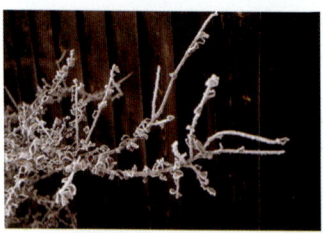

Time for myself ... Why is it I find it so hard to take time for myself? Time to be, rather than time to do. And often what is urgent, elbows its way to the forefront of my day and the important gets trampled in the rush. Teach me the art of creating islands of stillness, in which I can absorb the beauty of everyday things: clouds, trees, a snatch of music ... Impress upon your mind that there is more to life than packing every moment with activity, and help me to pencil in some part of my day with quietness.

Mark's GC, *Take Time To Just Be*

Take a moment to reflect: are you enslaved by addictions or negative thoughts? What is your energy level? Can you improve it?

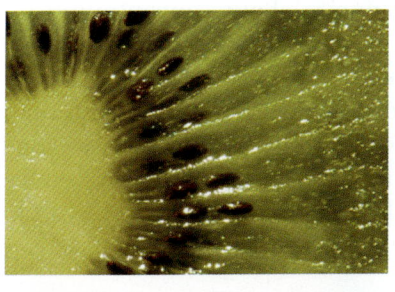

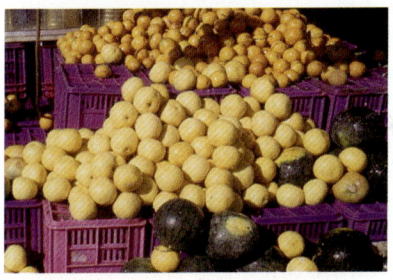

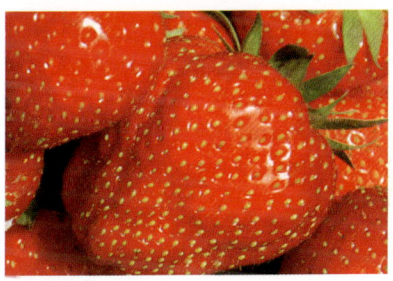

You didn't think when you got up this morning that this would be the day your life would change, did you? But it's going to happen because the only thing that stands between you and grand success in living are these two things: getting started and never quitting! You can solve your biggest problem by getting started, right here and now.

Robert H. Schuller, *Begin It Now*

Eat to Live, Not Live to Eat

It is thought that approximately one third of all cancers may be linked with diet. This section is about concentrating on what constitutes a healthy, balanced diet for life and not just for the duration of your cancer and its treatment.

Nutrition is about eating wholesome foods that nourish your mind, body and spirit. A nurturing diet encompasses foods that replenish the body with vital energy, instead of draining energy in the process of digestion. The following five steps will help you to assess how healthy your diet is:

Step one:

One third of your food at any meal should consist of fresh produce, such as fruit, vegetables, salads, as well as essential vitamins, pulses, protein, fibre, calcium and minerals.

Step two:

Try to get most of your protein from seafood and poultry. Red meat is also high in protein; however, it is best to limit red meat to maybe one meal each week.

Step three:

Dairy products and eggs are valuable in any diet, but choose low-fat dairy foods, like skimmed milk or small amounts of pure, natural butter which is far better for you than lots of the chemical margarines. Both have the same amount of calories.

Step four:

Avoid expensive processed foods; try home-made soup, vegetable casserole and beans as occasional alternatives to meat. It is also important to drink at least three litres of water a day, especially during your treatment. Dead cells and toxins are excreted from the body via the blood stream, so a good fluid intake helps to speed up the process of excreting toxins.

Step five:

The balance of good health means a reduced-salt, low-fat, high-fibre diet. Eat a variety of different foods. Remember, no food is a sin if it is only eaten occasionally. Healthy eating is not just about what you eat but how you prepare, eat and digest your food. It is important to pay attention to not only what you eat, but also how and where you eat.

Can you remember that china in your cupboard that you only use for best or when you have a dinner party? Don't you deserve the best each day? It's not just about appreciating the presentation of the food but the exquisite china! Set the table with flowers or candles, make the meal special – it is, after all, nutritional healing for you, to savour and enjoy.

Put on your favourite music, even if you live alone, because you deserve the best. If you eat with the family, use the time to love and appreciate each other, to share the experiences of the day. Let it be a time to talk and listen. If you are eating alone, appreciate the food, listen to the music and relax during this special time for yourself.

Food nourishes your body, but there are times when, for many reasons, we need to supplement our diet with vitamins and minerals. Even with a healthy diet, it is possible that nutritional excesses and deficiencies have occurred and this needs to be remedied. Additional vitamins and minerals can be helpful if you:

- are suffering from a viral infection

- smoke or someone else in your environment does

- live in a heavily populated area

- are under constant stress

During the winter months, additional vitamins and minerals should be taken if you:

- drink more than the recommended amount of alcohol each week

- are taking aspirin or regular medication

- spend a lot of time indoors

- are suffering from osteoporosis

- are having or have had chemotherapy, radiotherapy or surgery

What you eat should not cause you stress. A diet so rigid that your whole life revolves around it can increase anxiety and stress and therefore do more harm than good.

Patient experience:

The husband of a patient rang me one day asking for some advice. His wife had convinced herself that the cancer diet she was on must be adhered to at all times. Her husband and children found that they were spending every day buying fresh produce and preparing it for each meal. The diet had become an obsession and had taken over their life. Clearly, this was only adding to the family's stress and anxiety.

As a family, they had to sit down together, to explore and create enjoyable meals for all of them, to meet everybody's needs, not just the person with cancer.

This is not always easy. If you really feel that you want a piece of chocolate, a glass of wine or your favourite food, then have it as a treat and enjoy it. Food is your body's energy; you deserve the best you can afford to keep you healthy, to help you recover from treatment or just to maintain your body's wellness. Make it fun, make it special and make it with love as a gift to yourself.

There are many organisations and individuals who suggest that they have specific diets for cancer. You may wish to research or contact them directly to see if they are right for you. Always check with your specialist nurse, GP or oncologist as to what supplements or specific eating regimes you would benefit from. First, you need to assess what is causing the imbalance in your body. You can help to rebalance your body energy, either before, during or after your treatment for cancer, by:

- consuming energy-filled food from produce that is as fresh as possible in order to maintain physical energy

- eating fresh organic fruit and vegetables, together with complex carbohydrates such as potatoes, pasta, rice, wholemeal bread, beans and pulses, which are energy-providing foods

- taking a look at what chemical substances are in the food you eat and trying to eliminate them if your energy levels are low. Try to detoxify by drinking freshly squeezed fruit juices or smoothies. Check with your consultant if you are receiving chemotherapy prior to undergoing any changes in diet

- eliminating substances classified as energy thieves. You may be eating well, but you may not be getting total nutrition because you smoke, drink coffee, rely on alcohol or recreational drugs or are having chemotherapy or radiotherapy

- remembering to drink plenty of water a day. Add ice and a slice of lemon or lime to each glass of the recommended three litres a day to aid fast elimination of toxins in the body

- bearing in mind that during your chemotherapy/radiotherapy, you may find that your appetite changes and you may be aware of different tastes and smells related to a specific food. You may even want foods that previously you would not have eaten

- eating three meals each day during and after treatment may seem overwhelming. Eating little and often, such as healthy snacks of fruit and vegetables, may suit you better. If your mouth does not produce saliva, then try small pieces of pineapple to stimulate saliva production

- keeping the size of each portion of food small. It may be helpful to freeze small portions in an ice-cube tray, so that each snack is of something different

- bearing in mind that with the exception of green olive oil, all fats that line supermarket shelves have gone through processing, turning healing foods into killing foods. The fats in pork, beef, lamb, dairy and tropical nuts are natural and not synthetic or damaged by processing

- being aware that the two essential fats are omega-3 and omega-6, found in oily fish. Both are sensitive to destruction by light

- noting that excess sugar in our body is turned into hard fats, damaging teeth and feeding bacteria, yeast infections and cancer cells.

Of the fifty essential nutrients our bodies need, two come from fats and oils and the remaining forty-eight from vitamins, minerals and essential amino acids from proteins.

We are what we eat and it can influence your health in both a positive and a negative way, if we allow it. A balanced diet should be made up of a good mix of:

- fruit and vegetables (remember: five a day)

- complex carbohydrates

- proteins such as salmon, chicken and turkey and omega-3 oils.

Sometimes, carers become frustrated because what they prepare is often not eaten. If this is the case, both of you may want to consult with a dietitian and this could be arranged by your GP. A nurturing diet utilises foods that replenish the body with vital energy. Often, patients find certain foods highly aromatic and difficult to be around, causing nausea. This may change daily and make meal planning difficult. The size of the portions of food can be overwhelming, so use a small plate. You may find drinking plain water difficult, so try making fruit-flavoured ice cubes to keep your body hydrated, especially whilst receiving chemotherapy or radiotherapy.

Keep a wide range of foods in the house and always buy small sizes, to reduce waste. Don't get distressed about what to cook, keep mealtimes a fun time. Instead of breakfast, lunch and dinner, have five or six small snacks a day.

Things do not change; we change.
Henry David Thoreau, *Begin It Now*

Take a moment to reflect: which of the five factors do you think you have to work on to achieve body wellness?

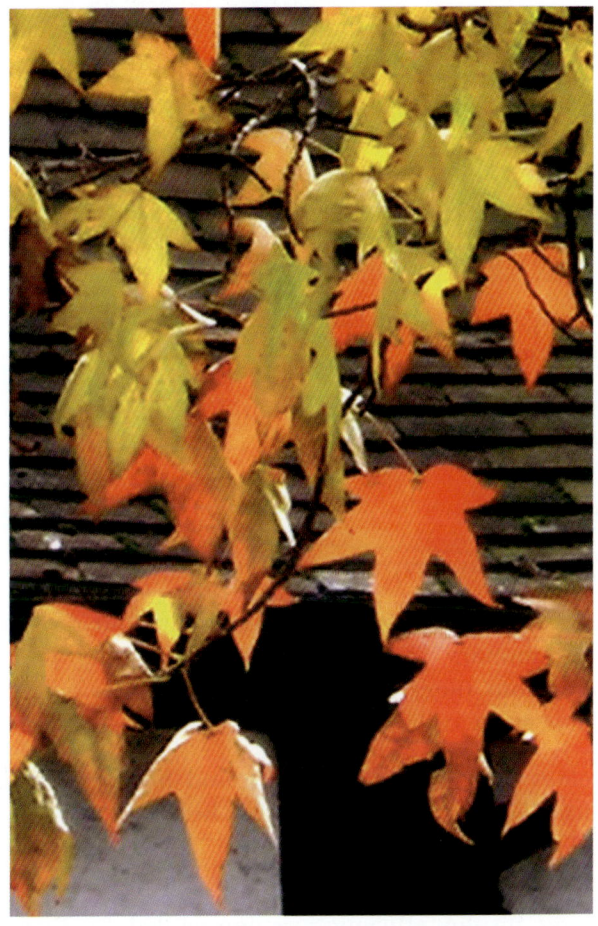

Intelligence highly awakened is intuition; which is the only true guide in life.

Krishnamurti, *Begin It Now*

Enjoyable Exercise

Enjoyable exercise helps you to maintain a balanced energy that strengthens your body and calms your mind. Exercise revitalises your body, stimulates your healing force and inspires inner confidence and firm resolve. Enjoyable exercise should engage you in some form of vigorous physical activity, which causes you to sweat or breathe faster for twenty minutes, at least three times a week. Exercise is crucial for good health. Examples of exercise from everyday activities:

- if you're able, take the stairs rather than the lift

- if you love walking, do it regularly

- if exercise or playing sport has not always appealed in the past, give it a try

- enjoy yoga as exercise rather than relaxation or why not try t'ai chi?

- if your mobility is restricted, then do some stretching and flexing exercises sitting down

Exercise:

- can help you to overcome stress or depression

- increases your endurance physiologically, your respiration and pulmonary functioning and your lung capacity, allowing four times the normal amount of oxygen to be available at the cellular level

- decreases resting blood pressure and heart rate, raising abnormally low blood pressure and heart rate

- reduces natural diuretic fluid retention problems

- increases insulin efficiency recommended in Type Two diabetics

- increases circulation to the capillaries which help to feed muscles and other tissues

- helps to maintain bone strength and posture

- provides the stimulus to keep bone mass at a high level, minimising the likelihood of osteoporosis

- increases substances vital to wound repair

- reduces muscle wasting

- reduces pain (arthritis) and lowers blood pressure

- increases the release of endorphins (natural painkiller)

- is a natural antidepressant, which has a calming effect on the mind, significantly reducing anxiety and contributing to better sleep

- a fifteen-minute brisk walk produces more relaxation at the muscular level than a tranquilliser

- decreases stress-related fatigue

- builds self-esteem and confidence

- increases stimulation to the right hemisphere of the brain for greater creativity

- is a preventative factor for cancer

- reduces obesity, which is implicated in cancer and other life-threatening conditions

- raises the core body temperature which debilitates and kills abnormal cells

- increases immune system cell production through increased Beta-endorphins

- increases resistance to diseases and infection

- reduces the immune system compromise response to emotional assaults such as cancer diagnosis

- dissipates substances such as cortisol and catecholamine, which are associated with depression of the immune system

Whatever your ability, make exercise enjoyable. You can exercise both on your own and with others. Remember: you do not have to achieve Olympic standards, unless you really want to. Alternate the type of exercise. Some ideas of the level of exercise you might expect to achieve are listed below:

Light exercise that can be fun:

- walks of 2 miles or more

- light DIY

- table tennis

- miniature golf

- social dancing

- bowling

- occupations not entirely sedentary

- t'ai chi

Moderate exercise that can be fun:

- long walks of over 2 miles at brisk or fast pace

- swimming

- tap dancing

- line dancing

- heavy DIY

- heavy gardening

- heavy housework

- active but not vigorous occupations

Vigorous exercise that can be fun:

- hillwalking at a brisk pace

- running/jogging

- football/tennis/squash

- aerobics

- cycling

- exercise that makes you breathless and makes you sweat

- ice skating

- paintballing ... the list is endless!

Take a moment to reflect: what activity did you do today, just for fun?

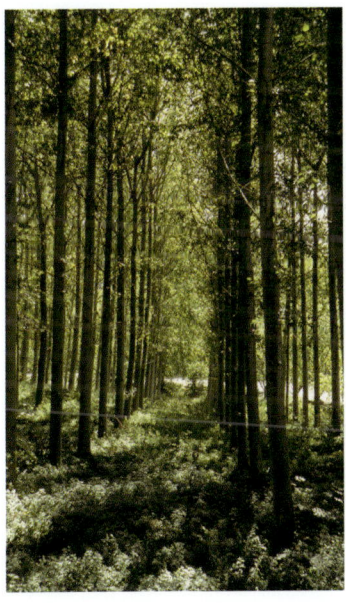

Some people walk in the rain, others just get wet!
Roger Miller, *Bag of Jewels*

Why and How to Exercise

We all have many reasons why we don't exercise, but if we are to stay healthy we need to motivate ourselves or join an activity with a friend, making it enjoyable and fun. Our mind will play tricks and always give us a negative reason not to exercise, but we need to change that negative into a positive action:

Negative reason: not enough time can be fitted into normal daily life to exercise

Positive action: cycling to work, walking to local shops

Negative reason: exercise makes you tired

Positive action: exercise makes you less tired; why don't you try it and see?

Negative reason: exercise can be dangerous

Positive action: danger can easily be avoided and it is more dangerous not to exercise

Negative reason: exercise makes you stiff

Positive action: activity need not be sport, try gardening or walking the dog

Negative reason: a dislike of sport

Positive action: activity need not be sport

Negative reason: a dislike of group activity

Positive action: you can be active alone

Negative reason: a dislike of activity alone

Positive action: you can be involved in group activity if you want

Negative reason: no money

Positive action: walking costs nothing, skipping costs just a few pence

Once you have chosen your enjoyable exercise, remind yourself why you are doing it. Is it because you need to change your lifestyle? Is it part of your journey to health? I would now like to address some basic tips on staying safe while exercising:

Physical activity safety code:

It is important for you to be safe when undertaking exercise. Always check with your doctor if you are uncertain about the exercise you have chosen:

- The benefits of physical activity come from a regular, graduated programme. Erratic participation in vigorous activity is potentially hazardous. When you decide what sort of physical activity you will take up, make sure that it will be possible for you to maintain regular participation and build it slowly.

- There is nothing to be gained from overexertion. Begin slowly and build up gradually, with a gentle progression to extend your limits.

- Warming up and cooling down for periods of about ten minutes each are necessary before and after vigorous exercise. A few simple stretches and loosening exercises are advisable even before a brisk walk. Proceed with a slow walk following your simple warm-up.

- Vigorous activity should never be stopped abruptly. A short period of moderate and then light activity and gentle stretching helps to avoid stiffness.

- Wear suitable clothing and protective equipment if necessary, paying particular attention to good footwear.

Whether you choose to exercise in your own home alone or with a group, whether you decide to explore t'ai chi or yoga, the most important thing is that you do something that you enjoy. If you don't then you will not be committed to it. Exercise should be a part of normal life. Explore new forms of exercise, experience them and discover what is right for you. Perhaps one of the best forms of exercise is walking, not just because of its workout for the body but for the emotional gain. If you choose to walk in a favourite park or area, you can do so on a daily basis and enjoy the changing face of nature as you watch the seasons come and go.

Be aware of the brightness and freshness of spring, with the colours and growth of new plants. As summer approaches, the hot, lazy days change the natural landscape. Smell fresh-cut grass and see the corn and wheat fields, the summer flowers and the beauty of the insects. Lie down in that field as you did as a child and stare at the blue sky and daydream. Then experience the rustle of autumn, with its rich golden and copper colours. It will encourage you to put on your walking shoes and kick up the crisp leaves as they fall and collect the cones, conkers and acorns. When winter approaches, wrap up warm and see the beauty in the early morning frost and the robins foraging. Go out in the snow, throw a snowball, make a snowman, walk on the white carpet and trace your footsteps as you move forward. Walking takes you back to the beauty of nature. See it, smell it, feel it, touch it, in all its beauty.

> Be willing to do what your soul directs you to do if you
> want to create what you are asking for.
>
> Sanyana Roman, *Bag of Jewels*

Take a moment to reflect: ask yourself how many times during the past four weeks you have taken any sort of physical activity at all, including walking, that lasted twenty minutes or more.

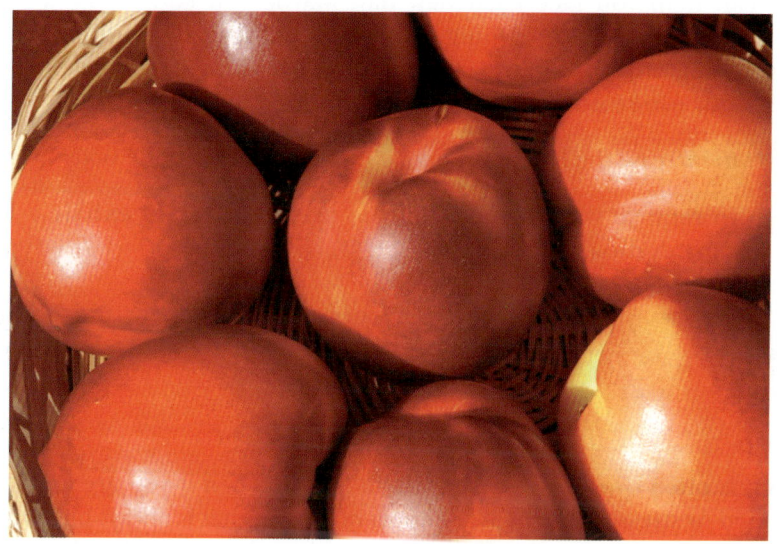

Don't evaluate your life in terms of achievements, trivial or monumental, along the way ... Instead, wake up and appreciate everything you encounter along the path. Enjoy the flowers that are there for your pleasure. Tune in to the sunrise, the little children, the laughter, the rain, and the birds. Drink it all in ... there is no way to happiness; happiness is the way.

Dr Wayne W. Dryer, *Taking Time to Just Be*

Body Fatigue

Rest allows us to be involved with something that is enjoyable and often creative as well. It allows our breathing and physical body to relax at a deeper level. The mind is quietened from everyday thoughts, as we are immersed in relaxing pursuits.

Think about the last time you really relaxed. What was it that you were doing? How did it make you feel? Breathing is a great way to relax and can help you face each new day. Maybe you could take a walk around your garden, breathing deeply and relaxing all the time. While undergoing chemotherapy or radiotherapy it is important to breathe deeply for two reasons:

- to increase the intake of circulating oxygen around the body

- to remove waste products from the body as you exhale carbon dioxide

Rest allows you to channel your energy into repairing and healing your body.

Sleep

Sleep is often one of the first areas to be disturbed if you are anxious, worried or stressed. If you are the sort of person that is always on the go, you are using all your energy for your activities. If you are sleeping, then your body's energy can be utilised for repair and healing. Through our dreams we often bring solutions and answers from our subconscious into our conscious mind. If you are having difficulty sleeping run through the list below to see if anything will help:

- establish a pattern – avoid stimulants such as tea and coffee after 8.00 p.m.

- check your medication, particularly if you are taking steroids, as it is important to take these before 6.00 p.m.; otherwise they will affect your sleeping

- a massage for twenty minutes or ten minutes of yoga before bed will help you relax and let go of the thoughts of the day

- do not underestimate the relaxing effects of making love with your partner

- add three drops of sweet orange and three drops of lavender essential oils to a vaporiser fifteen minutes before bed. Always ensure you have extinguished the candle flame before you fall asleep

- herbal remedies such as valerian may be extremely useful for sleep problems; this herb relieves anxiety and helps to improve sleep quality. Always check with your oncologist before taking any herbal remedies

- what you eat can affect your ability to sleep; avoid sugary snacks or a heavy meal after 8.00 p.m.

- to maintain your blood sugar overnight, you may find a small bowl of cereal may help you to sleep

- choose foods rich in the amino acid tryptophan, such as fish, seaweed, dates, oats, eggs, avocados, almonds and yogurt

- if you go to sleep easily but wake up in the early hours of the morning feeling anxious and restless, it might be worth trying a homeopathic remedy

- if you wake early and cannot get back to sleep, or you have been dreaming, keep a notebook next to your bed and either write down your dream or what is going on in your head that is keeping you awake. Don't think about it; just write as it comes naturally and then try to return to bed and sleep

- to create a good flow of energy in your bedroom, follow one of the feng shui solutions, which is to cover any mirrors that show your reflection while you are in bed. Mirrors attract energy and can cause restless nights

- decorate your bedroom with soft, restful colours; make it a room that is peaceful and calm

- ensure the bedroom is uncluttered and conducive to rest and sleep

- if you need to buy a new bed, choose a wooden one rather than a metal one, as it is less likely you will be affected by electromagnetic stress

- ensure your bedroom temperature is just right, not too hot or too cold

It is normal to feel anxious before you have surgery, radiotherapy or chemotherapy and sleep may be disturbed. However, remember your deep breathing, relaxing into every breath. Also, try a relaxation or visualisation technique as you go to bed; it will help you to relax and fall asleep. As a last resort, a teddy bear to cuddle has also been known to help.

Give yourself permission to relax now, for thirty minutes!

Take a moment to reflect: can you remember the last time you really relaxed? Where were you and what were you doing that helped you relax?

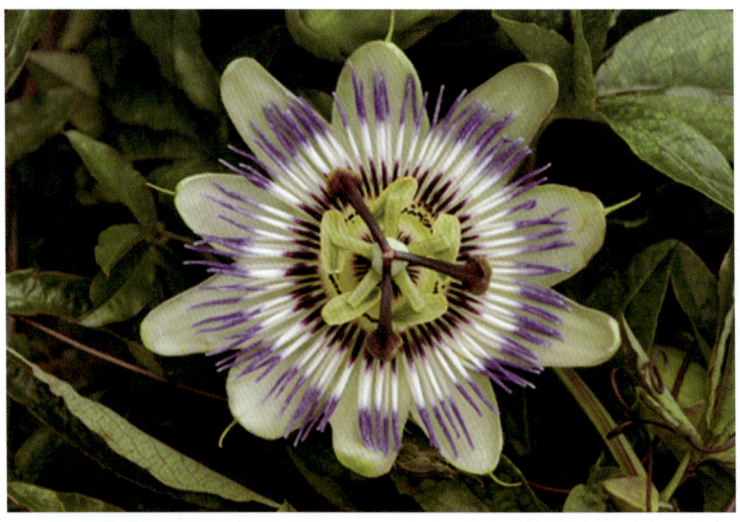

If you can spend a perfectly useless afternoon in a perfectly useless manner, you have learned how to live.
Lin Yutang, *Taking Time To Just Be*

A healthy immune system

The World Health Organisation determines health as a state of complete physical, mental, emotional and social well-being, not merely the absence of disease or infirmity. A strong immune system makes you invincible and able to lead a healthy, active and long life. Your immune system is your personal medical team, there to protect you, heal you and enable you to respond in a crisis and always be on call. In order to remain well, you need to look after your immune system. Your immune system has many enemies, some of which you cannot always avoid. The more enemies that attack at any one time, the less effective your immune system is at beating and destroying them. Immune system enemies include:

- smoke

- stress

- accidents

- pollution

- genetic defects

- food additives

- pesticides

- drugs

- lack of exercise

- radiation

- being overweight

- infection

- incorrect balance of nutrition

- being underweight

- pessimistic attitude to life

- inadequate vitamin and mineral balance

- undergoing radiotherapy or chemotherapy

- undergoing surgery

The list is daunting. However, you should acknowledge factors that can weaken your immune system and then positively look at how you can boost it. We all need a healthy immune system because it:

- fights off viruses, bacteria and other common and rare organisms

- helps to destroy and eliminate cancer cells following treatment

- aids elimination of your body's toxins every day

- provides protection from chemicals, pollution and radiation

- can increase allergy or autoimmune diseases if it deteriorates or loses its function

- determines how fast you age

An unhealthy immune system means you are:

- unwell for longer, more frequently and more seriously if undergoing treatment for cancer

- it is essential that you boost your immune system if you are receiving chemotherapy and radiotherapy, as they do not only kill cancer cells but also normal cells.

- a healthy immune system needs to regenerate between treatment cycles; this will reduce side effects and also make you feel well enough to tackle the next treatment

We may never reach that ideal standard of an undistinguishable balance of mind, body and spirit, which means that most of us are in various stages of energy imbalance most of the time. However, we are capable of striving for excellence and by maintaining your immune system in the best possible condition, you can use your body's defences and energy to fight cancer. Our mind can also help us through imagery, to mobilise our fighter cells to destroy the cancer cells or the toxic effect of the treatment.

Take a moment to reflect: what immune system enemies do you have?

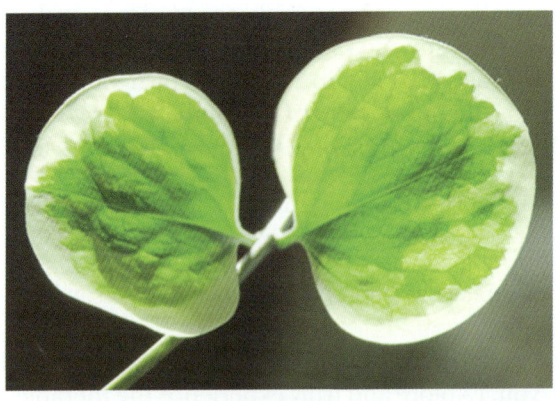

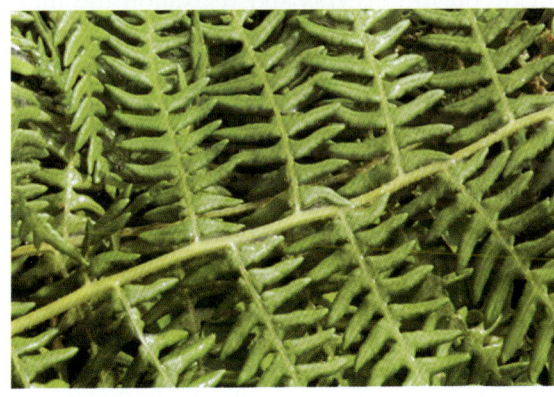

He who knows others is wise.
He who knows himself is enlightened.

Lao-Tzu, *Bag of Jewels*

Cancer and Complementary Therapies

By exploring complementary therapies you can discover new ways of coping with cancer. I am sure you are very aware of times when your physical body is stressed, but it is important to identify where the tension is and perhaps look at some of the complementary therapies available to you that may provide relaxation and reduce muscle tension.

Allow yourself the opportunity to explore and experience a complementary therapy. No one therapy is right for everyone. Discover what works for you, what fits in with your own values and beliefs and what gives you the most benefit. Perhaps the two most important elements when considering complementary therapies are:

- that you feel that the practitioner's intent and presence are right for you, and

- that a therapeutic relationship exists between you and the therapist

Establishing a relationship with others is part of achieving harmony and being true to you. Explore and truly experience the therapies with an open mind and decide on the benefits and relaxation the therapy gives you. Many cancer centres now provide some complementary therapies; others will be available on a fee-paying basis. Always ask to see the practitioner's qualifications and ask what professional organisation registers them fit for practice/insurance. Always remember to let the practitioner know if you are on medication or currently having chemotherapy or radiotherapy. Look at the options and see what is right for you. Ask your hospital if they provide this service or if they could recommend a practitioner. Always check with your oncologist before starting any therapy.

Reflexology:

This is a specialised form of massage of the feet and hands, performed to detect and correct imbalances in the body that may be causing ill health. It is, however, much more than a simple massage. Modern reflexology stems mainly from the work early in the twentieth century of two Americans, Dr Fitzgerald and Eunice Ingham. It was Dr Fitzgerald who first proposed the theory that the body is divided into ten equal zones that extend the full length of the body. Stimulation of the foot or hand in one zone affects other parts of the body in the same zone. Reflexology can also be deeply relaxing.

Ayurveda:

This is the ancient healing science of India. It embraces a code of healthy living and a natural treatment system in which purity of mind is necessary for encouraging physical health through the strength and flow of prana – the vital life force.

Ayurveda aims to eliminate the root cause of disease by providing moderation and balance between human beings and their environment. All aspects of living are involved in inspiring prana to create harmony within the body, mind and spirit. Thus, ethics, emotions and devotion assume equal importance with climate, good nutrition and exercise. In Ayurveda, one or more of six tastes – sweet, sour, bitter, pungent, astringent and salty – is used to describe the healing properties of different herbs and fruits.

Relaxation therapies:

These consist of therapeutic massage, relaxation techniques, aromatherapy, guided visualisation and imagery and they are all good for calming the body. Relaxation therapies can also help you to view the situation more positively; people with an upbeat approach to cancer have a better chance of beating it.

Types of Massage:

Massage is an excellent way to relax mind and body and so bring relief from everyday stresses and strains. Through touching and stroking, a sense of calmness and balance can be restored. A body massage can enhance general health and well-being. It can coax tension from muscles, ease stiff joints, provide healthy circulation of the blood and stimulate lymphatic drainage, to encourage the elimination of waste products from the body.

Shiatsu:
This is an ancient form of pressure-point massage. It is based on the principles of the Chinese discipline of acupuncture, applying pressure to key points, with the purpose of balancing your life energy.

Therapeutic massage:
This comforting form of massage consists of soothing strokes and gentle touch using only 'carrier oil', such as almond oil, and is now in wide use in both conventional and

complementary medicine. In recent years it has been shown to benefit the mind and body of people with cancer. It is essential that you inform the practitioners of any nut allergies you may have as some carrier oils contain nut essence.

Biodynamic massage:
This therapy combines massage with elements of physical exercise and psychological development.

Aromatherapy:

This is the use of essential oils from plants to enhance general health and well-being. It can be used in a variety of ways. Each essential oil has its own characteristic aroma and profile of therapeutic properties. Some oils are soothing and relaxing, others have a stimulating and invigorating combination. Essential oils are highly concentrated; therefore, only a few drops should be used.

Essential oils should not be put directly onto skin but should be mixed with carrier oil, such as almond, grape seed, wheat germ, jojoba or olive oil, and then used as a massage oil. If you are receiving chemotherapy or radiotherapy, check with your consultant before using massage oils on the skin.

Leisure
What is this life, if full of care,
We have no time to stand and stare?–
No time to stand beneath the boughs,
And stare as long as sheep and cows:
No time to see, when woods we pass,
Where squirrels hide their nuts in grass:
No time to see, in broad daylight,
Streams full of stars, likes skies at night:
No time to turn at Beauty's glance,
And watch her feet, how they can dance:
No time to wait till her mouth can
Enrich that smile her eyes began?
A poor life this if, full of care,
We have no time to stand and stare.

W. H. Davies, *101 Poems*

Take a moment to reflect: did you make time today to find out more about complementary therapies? Have you made an appointment for a consultation with a complementary therapy practitioner?

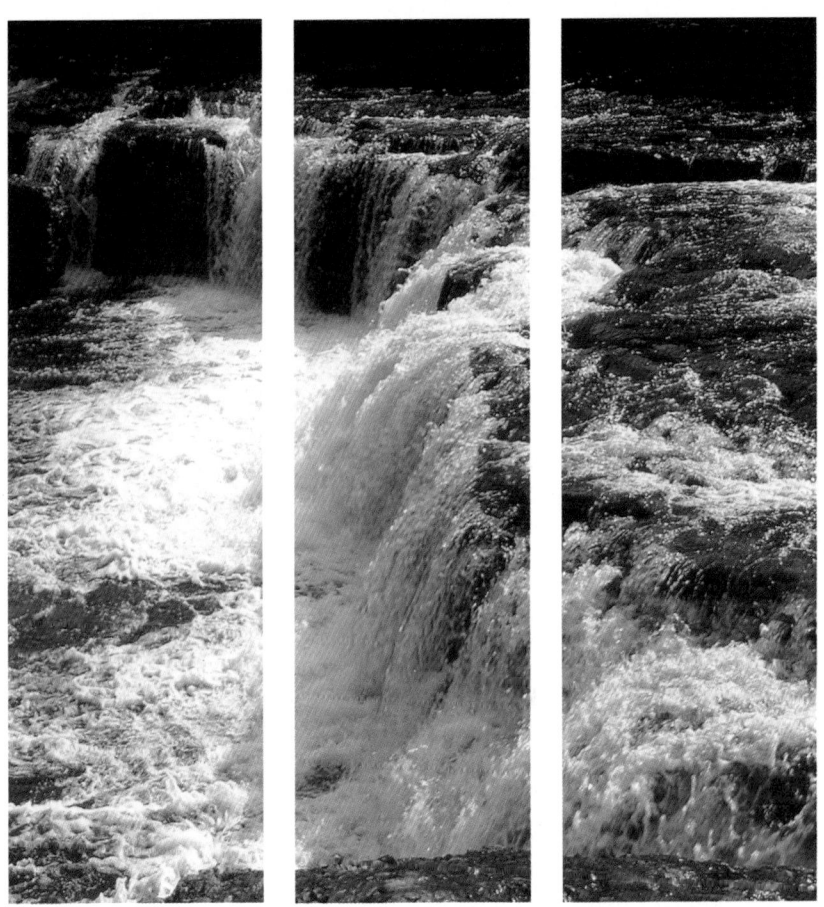

To change one's life: Start immediately,
do it flamboyantly, no excuses!

William James, *Begin It Now*

Deep-breathing exercise:

Because of the nature of life in the twenty-first century there may be times when you find it very hard to relax and let go of your tension. One of the best ways to begin to relax is to focus all thoughts on your breathing, which is often shallow when stressed. You need to change to deep-breathing exercises to help with muscle tension.

One of the aims of these exercises is to retrain our bodies to breathe fully using the diaphragm, the muscle that is responsible for causing the lungs to inflate and take in oxygen. When we shallow breathe we forget to use the full capacity of the lung, which is essential if we are to take in enough oxygen.

Normal healthy cells require oxygen to function. Oxygen deficiency in cells could be a major contributory factor in healthy cells mutating and becoming cancerous. Many recognised carcinogens are known to inhibit or restrict oxygen circulation in the body.

Body relaxation:

Prepare for relaxation by finding a quiet place, where you will not be disturbed by the telephone, family or conversation. Within this quiet place find something to lie or sit on and make yourself comfortable. A blanket or a pillow may also help, together with or without some gentle background music. Ensure your head is comfortable and supported.

Breathing:

Start to be aware of your breathing. Concentrate on breathing in and breathing out. Feel your breath slowing, flowing in and out. It may be that you want to count as you inhale – one – two – exhale – three – four – or perhaps you find repeating a phrase like 'I am at peace', 'I am calm', 'I am relaxed' more helpful. Find out what is right for you. There is no right way, only what works for you. When your breathing is relaxed, you can begin to relax the body.

Relaxing the body:

Some people find it helpful to systematically work through the body from head to toe or vice versa; tighten and relax each group of muscles. Become aware of your toes on your right foot. Tighten them and hold it, then let them relax. Then focus on the ankle. Tighten it and hold it before letting your right ankle feel loose and relaxed. Continue moving up to your right calf, thigh, buttock, etc. Feel the tension, hold and relax. Continue to focus on all areas of your body, first the right side and then the left side.

When you have worked through the body, just notice what it feels like to be relaxed and calm. Say the words 'relaxed and calm', 'relaxed and calm'. At this point, you can stay physically relaxed for however long you choose. When you are ready to end the session, bring yourself back to your quiet room, and slowly open your eyes. Take in your surroundings, move your position and notice how refreshed and alert you feel.

Visualisation:

Once your body is relaxed you may want to work through a visualisation process. You can use this one or choose one of your own.

Let your mind gently wander; think of going for a day out in the country. Where would you go? Where is your special place? Visualise yourself arriving and looking around. Notice the colours, the light and the patterns of shade. What sounds can you hear? Are they near or far away? Is there music? What are the sounds of nature saying? Notice the season. Is it spring, summer, autumn or winter? What temperature is it? Perhaps there might be a cool breeze that you can feel. What can you smell that is pleasant and comforting? Enjoy the moment.

It is up to you if you want to stay there or move gently down a path, or round a corner, or over a hill. This is your special place – stay there as long as you wish. Feel the calm, the peace. Breathe in the beauty of nature. Notice how completely relaxed you are.

When you're ready, slowly bring yourself back into the room and open your eyes. Notice your surroundings and gently stretch or slowly move your position. In your own time, be aware of feeling refreshed and re-energised.

When you are waiting for a hospital appointment or to see your consultant, try deep breathing and visualise a place you would much rather be, until your name is called for the consultation. Did it reduce your stress during the consultation?

Yoga:

This aims to improve overall health and well-being by stimulating your inner healing forces that create a pathway to wellness. Yoga postures strengthen, relax and improve the flexibility of muscles and joints and they help maintain movement in the upper body, shoulders and arms. Yoga not only improves your physical well-being but it also increases longevity. Through physical postures one obtains a harmony and through breathing and concentration one finds tranquility. Yoga has the following advantages:

- improves oxygenation of the blood

- exercises the mind through physical movements

- produces reserves of energy

- relaxes the mind

- helps maintain good body posture

- improves the circulation of blood and lymph

- non violent and peaceful and has no age limit

The benefits of yoga are enhanced if you follow your routine with a period of relaxation, allowing you the full benefit of restoring your mind, body and spirit.

To help you develop your own skills and yoga postures, choose a teacher who understands the reasons why you have chosen yoga. Decide if you want to learn as a member of a group or if you wish to have individual sessions. Only you will know what is right for you. There are many different schools of yoga and it may help to find out about each one or visit a class and speak to the instructor. A few of the yoga schools are briefly described below:

Hatha Yoga – now usually understood to be the form that emphasises physical posture and position (or asana) and breathing control techniques (or pranayama).

Raja Yoga – now regarded as primarily involving meditation, being based on the mental aspects of yoga, rather than on the physical asana.

Ashtanga Yoga – continues elements of hatha and raja yoga. The basis of the practice is the linking of strenuous hatha positions and postures into almost continuous movement, while using the mind to affect breathing control.

Kundalini Yoga – traditionally referred to as the 'coiled serpent' at the base of the spine. It is a process of awakening the dormant subtle energy, so that it moves up the spine to the head, activating major energy centres (chakras), and as it does so ultimately causing changes in consciousness.

Tantric Yoga – based on texts that explain the importance of awakening the kundalini force. One part of tantric yoga seeks to use sexual pleasure as a means of heightened awareness, but classic tantric yoga also includes asana and pranayama of hatha yoga.

T'ai chi:

T'ai chi is often translated as meaning 'supreme ultimate', but a much more accurate translation is 'supreme energy' and this gives us a much better insight into its true nature. Often seen or described as a slow, gentle exercise, a moving meditation used for relaxation or an ancient practice used for healing and improving vitality, t'ai chi is all of these and more.

T'ai chi was originally a Chinese martial art whose origins are thousands of years old. It is known as an internal art, which means it focuses on using inner power or internal energy, rather than brute strength and physical techniques.

Energy is in us and around us in many different forms and states. Most of the time we are not aware of it or how we interact with it, but once we begin to become aware of it and experience it for ourselves, we can begin to realise how we can affect energy and how energy affects us.

The Chinese have been studying energy for many thousands of years and their systems of healing, martial arts and philosophy are all based around their understanding of energy. The whole of t'ai chi is based upon energy (chi) – understanding and utilising physical movement and posture, breathing, meditation, psychological approach and mental focus – with the purpose of utilising the body's natural energy system and the energy that is all around us. T'ai chi can be used for the following:

- increasing health and vitality

- relaxation

- healing

- exercise

- self-defence

- spiritual development

Traditional Chinese medicine:

Chinese medicine regards good health as the result of a perfectly balanced interplay between opposing yet complementary forces. All life contains such forces, which are enshrined in the principles of yin and yang. The essential energy of life – its vital force, chi – is believed to peak when yin and yang are in harmony not only within the patient's body, but also in the patient's life as a whole. The effectiveness of acupuncture and herbal medicine, which lies at the heart of traditional Chinese medicine, is based on their ability to balance yin with yang and encourages the steady flow of chi.

Chinese philosophy:

The Chinese believe that from the great void of darkness (yin) came light and life (yang); the active male is born from yin, the passive female from yang. It also sees life as a continuous cycle in which yin and yang are always interacting.

Chinese principles of energy:

The Chinese believe that there is a vital force or energy that permeates everything and is essential for life. The Chinese call this 'chi', which means energy. All living things need chi to flow in order to remain healthy and alive and it is necessary to have a constant replenishment of this energy.

Feng shui:

This is the ancient Chinese art of balancing energies, by integrating people, buildings and landscapes to create a harmonious whole. Only when balance and harmony are achieved can the 'chi', the energy or life force of the universe, flow freely, resulting in good health, happiness and prosperity. Correcting bad feng shui is considered just as much a part of the healing process as prescribing herbs or applying acupuncture.

Acupuncture:

This originated in China and is a way of adjusting the body's 'life energy' ('chi') flow. It includes the insertion of needles into selected acupuncture points, along the meridians (energy pathways) of the body. Each meridian has a specific effect on each body system or organ. Acupuncture can be used to relieve symptoms as well as to promote general health and well-being.

Inserting slender needles along known lines of energy called meridians removes impediments, to allow the vital life force 'chi' to flow freely again. Acupuncture can increase energy levels and it enhances your sense of well-being. If you are considering acupuncture, ask your oncologist if your blood count is OK for this treatment.

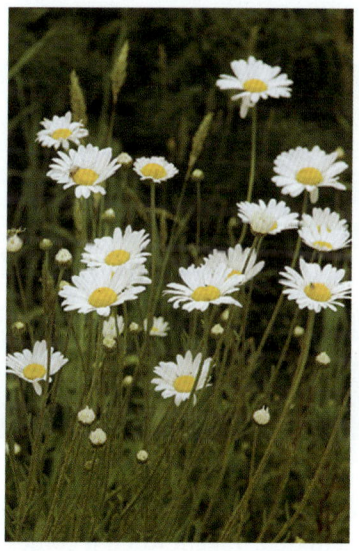

Always leave enough time in your life to do something that makes you happy, satisfied, even joyous.
That has more of an effect on economic well-being than any other single factor.

Paul Hawken, *Begin It Now*

Take a moment to reflect: it is said that we learn something new every day! What did you learn today? Was it about you or about others? What can you do to release your life from its daily hustle and bustle? What can you let go and what will you replace it with?

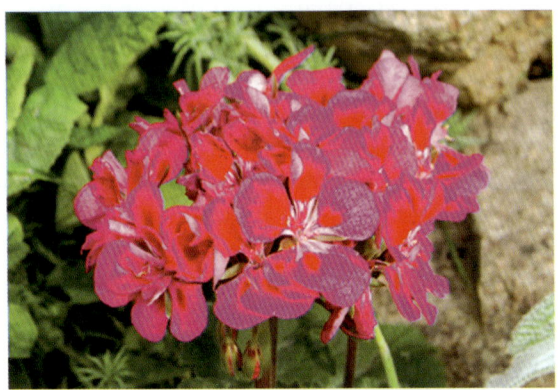

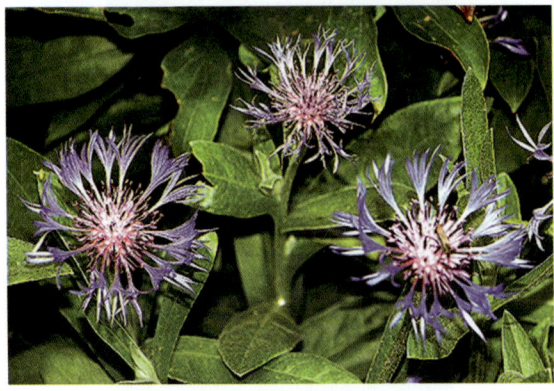

In the bustle of life, in the pressure of decisions, peace has become a luxury. Take it when it comes and cherish it. It gives you time to breathe. It gives you rest and a hope for life.

Pam Brown, *Taking Time to Just Be*

Energy Therapies

Reiki:

Reiki is the Japanese word for 'universal life energy' and it is pronounced 'ray kee'. It is a form of healing, based on tapping into the unseen flow of energy that is in all living things. The purpose of reiki is to work for the 'highest good'. It connects with the force of unconditional love, which transcends time and space.

Treatment by a reiki practitioner is intended to promote physical, emotional and spiritual well-being. It is a non-invasive form of healing and it is also deeply relaxing. Clients lie fully clothed while the practitioner's hands are placed over specific parts of the body, in line with the seven chakras:

1st Chakra	Root (Red)
2nd Chakra	Sacral (Orange)
3rd Solar Plexus	Lower Abdomen (Yellow)
4th Heart	Centre of Chest (Green)
5th Throat	Throat/Neck (Blue)
6th Brow	Forehead (Third Eye) (Indigo)
7th Crown	Top of the Head (Violet)

Reiki does not involve changing your religious beliefs and it can be used to heal yourself or others. Reiki energy can also be projected to a distant place and it can also be used on plants and animals.

Polarity therapy:

This was developed by Dr Randolph Stone, an Austrian-born naturopath, chiropractor and osteopath, who also took an interest in the therapies and practices of oriental medicine and spirituality. Polarity therapy is a holistic form of healing based on Stone's belief that humans are predominantly spiritual beings, whose health and happiness depend upon the free flow of energy within their bodies.

The guiding principle is that energy moves between positive and negative poles, through the body's chakras. The therapist uses the sense of touch, over each chakra, to release any blocked energy that may cause you ill health and he or she also provides counselling to encourage a positive attitude. Clients are asked to commit themselves to taking responsibility for their own health. Gentle stretching movements and a variety of detoxifying diets are also recommended.

Homeopathy:

This is a holistic form of medicine that aims to help the body heal itself. It works on both short-term and long-term illnesses and ailments and the prevention of illness is as crucial to its philosophy as is the treatment.

The word 'homeopathy' simply means treating like with like. This means that a substance that causes symptoms of illness in a well person can also be used to cure similar symptoms when they result from illness. Homeopathy treats disease by administering extremely small quantities of remedies from animal, vegetable and mineral sources. These remedies bolster natural healing forces that have the power to neutralise the destructive forces of disease. Homeopathy can treat almost any complaint – physical and psychological – although its therapeutic benefit appears to be dependent on each individual. Whole person prescribing is probably the most important part of homeopathy.

Diagnosis is made by careful consideration of feelings, reactions and personality type, as well as physical symptoms, in order to construct a complete portrait of the patient. Remedies are formulated in different concentrations but – theoretically – all would produce the very symptoms they are prescribed to relieve if used in much larger quantities.

Healing herbs:

Herbs may be natural and can be powerful healing tools; however, they can become toxic if taken in excess. Therapies involving plants, flowers and nutritional elements are some of the oldest and perhaps easiest to understand of all therapies available to us.

The Chinese, Japanese, Indian and Native American cultures all have traditional systems of herbal medicine. The approaches vary, but there is one important governing principle: that of 'synergism', which maintains that the strength of the sum of parts is greater than the strength of individual parts. Herbalists therefore use plant parts in their entirety, rather than isolating the plant's chemically active constituents. They believe that the combination of each and every element of a plant forms its healing properties and that each element has a specific role within the body. The combination of elements also works to prevent harmful side effects. Herbs can sometimes be used to treat cancer and they can also help with the side effects of conventional treatments, such as digestive and bowel problems, insomnia, mood swings and depression. Many current medicines are made up of chemicals imitating active ingredients that were once found in the natural formulas of herbal remedies.

The whole area of herbs is fascinating and may be something you would want to find out more about in relation to your treatment and recovery.

Flower and tree therapy:

Remedies from flowers and trees are subtle 'elixirs' that are claimed to be able to help rekindle a feeling of mental and emotional, as well as physical, well-being. Some are claimed to bring relief and healing. Bouchardon's nine energetic tree oils have qualities that include:

birch	gentleness and reconciliation
fir	respiration and fluidity
hawthorn	being in the present
beech	being prepared to go further
wild rose	opening
pine	bringing in light and vitality
boxwood	freedom and continuity
walnut	responsibility and autonomy
broom	renewal

Bach therapies:

Edward Bach, the founder of modern flower essence therapy, pioneered a holistic treatment by using safe and natural remedies. Bach now produces a directory of sixty of the best-known healing flowers with brief descriptions, followed by their uses and possible restriction. Take care when using flowers internally and consult a qualified herbalist, a Bach flower therapist or a pharmacist.

Most people's first introduction to flower essence therapy, and the most well-known of Bach remedies, is Rescue Remedy. This emergency formula has proved to be helpful for all kinds of stressful situations. Most chemists stock Rescue Remedy.

Crystal and gem therapy:

Practitioners believe that gems and crystals placed around or on the body can focus and enhance healing energy. The seven chakras in the body are used in crystal healing and the crystal of the colour associated with each chakra is placed on the body.

Crystals can be used in several ways: they can be held or placed around the home to absorb negative energy and improve the atmosphere. Crystal therapy is said to work on many levels, to encourage healing and to reduce mental and physical problems. There are many crystals to choose from and they have different attributes. Uncut stones are believed to possess more energy. Some powerful crystals include: red jasper, amethyst, rose quartz, malachite and quartz.

Again, like any new therapy you are trying, read about it and find out if it could be of benefit to you. Seek a registered practitioner and have a consultation with the therapist, which is usually free, before committing to any new therapy. Your local library or Health Authority will not only have information about complementary therapies but also where they are available in your area.

Moving towards body wellness is now a choice you have!

Decide what you want, decide what you will exchange
for it. Establish your priorities and go to work.

H. L. Hunt, *Begin It Now*

Take a moment to reflect: do you care for all of the five elements that constitute body wellness? Can you see benefits for your mind and body health?

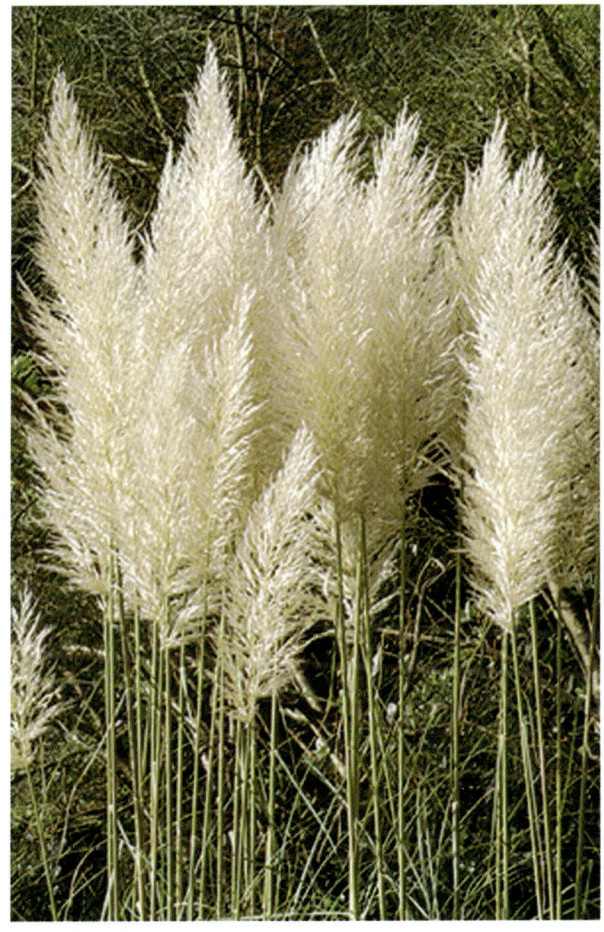

Plenty of people miss their share of happiness, not because they never found it, but because they did not stop to enjoy it.

William Feather, *Taking Time To Just Be*

Cancer and the Spirit

Faith is the bird that feels the light when the dawn is still dark.

Rabindranath Tagore, *Bag of Jewels*

Spiritual Wellness

Your body may have malignant cells, your mind may be defining you as a cancer patient, but the essential nature of who you are is beyond illness. We have looked at the mind and how to access and empower your positive energy and its mind and body connection. We have also looked at the body and how changing your lifestyle may turn a negative energy into positive action. In this section you can explore and assess your spirit energy in order for you to obtain holistic balance.

Defining the spirit as your third dimension is not always easy. Your spirit or essence is your true identity. It is the truth about you and it exists irrespective of time and setting. Your spirit energy, like mind and body energy, needs to be sustained, but how you chose to do that is unique to you. Your spirit is not your personality or your ego; your ego has no interest in your well-being. The only interest it has in keeping you alive is keeping itself alive, for it dies with your physical death. Until then it constantly whispers in your ear.

A state of wellness exists when your spirit, mind and body work in unison. Assessing the balance of your spirit requires you to draw upon your deepest healing resources. The five factors that determine your spirit's balance are:

Harmlessness:

To do no harm and to treat others as you would wish to be treated. In order to do this you need to be non-judgemental and help those in need. It means being a person that others trust, without exception.

Awareness:

Is about recognising you as a spiritual being. It means knowing that your body in interaction with your mind is the haven for your soul, while on earth. Awareness means undertaking everything you do with love.

Lovingness:

Is knowing that you are connected to all that is, was and ever will be. It comes with realising a divine presence in every living thing equally and impartially. This sacred knowledge is the breath of life.

Faith and devotion:

Is about being dutiful to your highest good and inspired by a sacred ideal. One needs to be constantly striving to live each moment in the inner light of unconditional love and truth.

Transcendence and joy:

Is about attaining and sustaining balance, harmony and peace of mind. It means being overwhelmed by the knowledge of your connection with the unconditional love and forgiveness from a higher power.

Each day of your life you will find new ways to recognise yourself as a spiritual being. Reflecting on your life's meaning and purpose will sustain your spirit. Signposts for maintaining your spiritual wellness include:

- loving one another, in every aspect of your life

- recognising that you have a sense of purpose and order that enables you to be guided through your spirit

- identifying your ideal and striving towards it

- recognising the sacred presence in every living thing

- knowing that goodness and love are the most powerful healers of all

- being willing to forgive

- seeing the joy in life

- fulfilling your potential

- staying in the here and now

- striving to not dwell on that which is past or live in fear of your future

- demonstrating a commitment to your community and a connectedness to the world

Assessing the wellness of the spirit reminds you of your deepest healing resources. Every fibre of your unique being is invested with a search for meaning and purpose, in order to eventually return to the source of life.

When you recognise yourself as a spiritual being having a human experience, you find ways to overcome feelings of separateness and isolation. Faith, love, forgiveness and surrender allow your spiritual energy to flow freely. This empowers the essential change needed to bring the energy of the spirit into perfect balance.

Take a moment to reflect: how do you sustain your spirit?

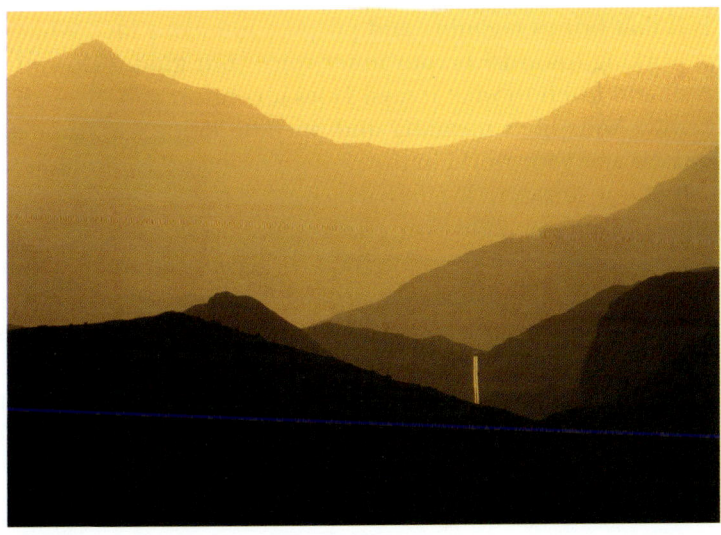

Spiritual Energy Balanced

Our entire universe is simply a wave of energy. From the finest atomic particle to the densest substance known, all life exists within this wave of energy that ebbs and flows in the great sea of existence. Your spirit is the source of all goodness. Being in a state of wellness opens your heart to the revelation that through love, you are connected to every living thing.

Love:

When you find ways to recognise yourself as a spiritual being the feeling of separateness and isolation can be overcome. Spiritual energy is about the unconditional love and forgiveness that we receive and give. Did you remember to forgive yourself today, for perhaps not loving yourself or others yesterday?

Here and now:

Each new day is yours. It is a gift, live it. Yesterday has gone and tomorrow may never arrive. Staying in the here and now is often difficult. We carry baggage from the past that we can't let go of or we hold on to fear and anxiety for the future, which stops us from seeing the beauty of today. Yes, you have cancer, but you also have the opportunity to live each day to the full.

Meaning and purpose:

What is it that brings meaning and purpose into your life? What ideals are you working towards? Is your inner voice your guide? Do you make time to sit and listen to what it says? Does it comfort you through times of difficulty? Your life's meaning and purpose helps you to be at one with yourself and your world in the present moment. Nature intends us to use all of our senses to live in balance.

Well-being is about fully living in the moment, while looking and feeling great. The extent to which you are 'sensory aware' is a measure of your capacity for life. Sensory awareness is your genetic heritage and a gift to be cherished. It has the ability to harmonise and express all aspects of your being.

The process of discovering your own unique truth will empower you to recognise a sacred presence in every living thing. The most powerful healers of all are forgiveness and love, of yourself and others.

Openness:

A feeling of openness signifies readiness to forgive yourself and others and let go of old negative thought patterns and beliefs. This moment is about opening up your spirit in order to explore and discover your own personal spiritual pathway.

Commitment:

This is about engaging with your health, well-being and personal growth and recognising that these are important and merit having energy and time devoted to them.

Awareness:

This is about knowing not merely what you are doing, but why you have chosen that option from all the others available. Move into your unique world of imagination, instinct and intuition. Establish contact with your inner healer by recognising the need to spend part of the day in silence, connected to your higher power.

Take a moment to reflect: what sustains you in times of trouble?

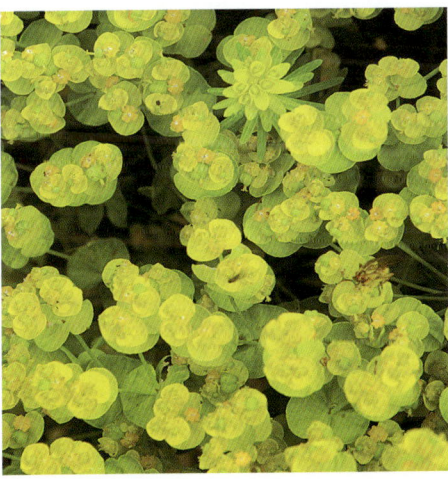

The great essentials to happiness in this life are something to do, something to love and something to hope for.

Joseph Addison, *Bag of Jewels*

111

Spiritual Stress

It is important to remember that spiritual stress relates in this instance to your spirit or essence, as distinct from earthbound body and mind. It is the domain of your intuition and integrity and your direct connection to a higher power. You may live by the text of organised religions or other articles of faith.

Articles of faith:

Paramahansa Yogananda, a great Indian sage, said that with the dawn of spiritual ambition we choose a chisel of wisdom to mould our life. Spend time contemplating the articles of faith enshrined in the following quotations:

Article 1   The unexamined life is not worth living. *Plato*

Article 2   We are what we repeatedly do. Excellence, then,
is not an act, but a habit. *Aristotle*

Article 3   Love is the beginning and the end, the alpha and
omega of existence. *Ethics of Judaism*

Article 4   Behind every blade of grass is its very own Angel
that forever whispers: grow ... grow ..., *Ethics of
Judaism*

Article 5   The most beautiful thing a person can do is to
forgive wrong, *Ethics of Judaism*

Article 6   Ask, and it shall be given you; seek, and you shall
find; knock, and it shall be opened unto you.
Testaments of Christianity

Article 7   Animosity does not eradicate animosity. Only by
loving-kindness is animosity dissolved. *Buddhist
Psalm*

Article 8   Wherever you turn, there is the face of God. *Koran*

Article 9   Start the day with love. Spend the day with love. Fill
the day with love. End the day with love. This is the
way to God, *Sathya Sai Baba*

The Christian faith – the Ten Commandments (abbreviated):

- Thou shall have no other Gods before Me

- Thou shall not make unto me any graven image

- Thou shall not take the name of the Lord thy God in vain

- Remember the Sabbath day, to keep it Holy

- Honour thy father and mother

- Thou shall not kill

- Thou shall not commit adultery

- Thou shall not steal

- Thou shall not bear false witness

- Thou shall not covet thy neighbour's house

Buddhism:

Buddhism is one of the most popular religions of today. Its teachings on kindness, simplicity and interconnectedness are attracting many people disenchanted with the world's all-pervading capitalism.

So how do you recognise spiritual stress? It is easy to recognise tension in muscles, caused by stress in our body, and the voice in our head that will not go silent because of psychological stress. Spiritual stress is about incongruence between what you think and what you feel, say or do. It is about telling that white lie, which comes back to haunt you. It is about doing or saying something that feels wrong to you and that remains with you however much you try to put it out of your mind. Spiritual stress is also about being something that you are not. It is about obeying your ego and living each day stroking your ego. Ultimately, your spirit will become smaller and smaller as your ego grows, but sooner or later something will happen which will bring into sharp focus the futility of your ego and the need to return to your original spiritual source.

Some cancer patients have said that when initially diagnosed, they in fact turned away from their faith or religion; they felt it had let them down. You often hear people say, 'How could God let something like this happen?' Sadly, bad things happen to good people and a life lived taking positive steps to maintain your body, mind and spirit in wellness often makes it difficult to understand why it has happened to you. Maybe it is about learning more about yourself than simply a matter of 'God letting it happen'. For all cancer patients it is the beginning of a personal journey, an opportunity to evaluate your life and make changes for the better.

Patient Experience:

A patient with lymphoma seemed reluctant to have further chemotherapy and each week she appeared more despondent and began to blame the doctors that the treatment was not working. On this particular day, whilst her blood was being taken, she told me that she was going to stop the treatment. She began to cry and revealed that she had only agreed to the treatment because it was what the family wanted and because she did not want to let them down. We talked about it for a while and she agreed to sit down with her family and her Macmillan nurse and tell them how she really felt. Her blood count was too low for treatment and I agreed to see her again in a week.

This patient was experiencing spiritual stress. She was having treatment not for herself but for the family, so she was not truly committed to the treatment and found that she could no longer keep up the pretence. She needed to make a decision about her treatment and commit to it. For this lady her family needed to hear what she really wanted to do.

The ultimate aim of spiritual practice is awakening, to know your true self, and your relationship with your 'higher power', whoever that may be. Gradually, the heart begins to open, fear and anger melt away, greed and jealousy dwindle, happiness and joy grow, love flourishes, peace replaces agitation, concern for others blossoms, wisdom matures and both the physical and psychological health improve.

Many patients found that their specific organised religion caused them stress when faced with cancer. Some felt that they had brought the cancer upon themselves or that the cancer was some kind of retribution for the way they had lived their life. When facing cancer it is important to have a faith that sustains your spirit during this difficult time; it is not the time for judgement.

Take a moment to reflect: do you experience spiritual stress?

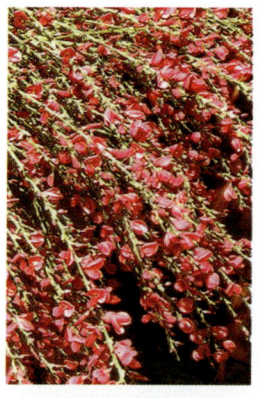

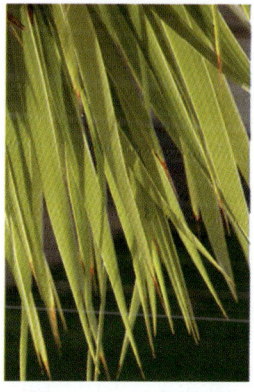

What you love is a sign from your higher self of what you are to do.

Sanyana Roman, *Bag of Jewels*

Sustaining the Spirit

Individuals need to know they are valued and that what they do is valued. We all need a place of peace and security as we all have spiritual needs of our own. Your spiritual dimension needs to connect to your own spiritual source on a daily basis, to keep your spiritual energy balanced. Some may say that they don't have a spiritual pathway and therefore they have little to sustain them in times of need. For balanced spiritual energy the essence of who you are is also based on your own values and beliefs. Do they empower you to allow you to:

- commit to positive affirmations to meet your mind's needs?

- listen to your intuition and wisdom to meet your body's needs?

- harness the sacred energy to sustain and meet your spirit's needs?

As the heart opens and the mind clears you finally find the most profound, the most meaningful and the most important discovery any human can make about themselves. It can:

- transform your motivation, reduce craving and help you to find your soul

- cultivate emotional wisdom, heal your heart and teach you how to learn to love

- help you to live ethically and feel good by doing good

- concentrate and calm your mind

- awaken spiritual vision, so that you may see clearly and recognise the sacred in all things

- cultivate spiritual intelligence, to enhance your life

- express your spirit, thought and action so that you may embrace generosity and joy through service to yourself and others

Patient Experience:

My surgery and treatment had finished and I thought I would be delighted and that I would be able to get back to normal life, whatever that is. But each day I felt something was niggling at me and I could not lay it to rest. One day I went for a walk and strolled into a church. I had allowed my faith to lapse when I was diagnosed and no longer felt a connection to my religion.

As I sat in the church, I realised that what was niggling at me was the fact that I had not been to Confession for several months and so I had an internal struggle going on inside me. I felt angry, vulnerable and empty, despite the fact that family and friends surrounded me. I asked the priest if he could find time to speak with me, which he did.

Some weeks later I realised that my anger and emptiness had disappeared, my soul felt lighter and I began to explore new avenues of spirituality applicable to me at the time. I had to take the time to face that struggle and work on sustaining my spirit. It is the template by which you live that walks beside you or carries you when you go through times of great difficulty. Spirituality is about having faith and putting your life in the hands of a higher power.

It may be that you want to research different faiths or to explore spirituality further and now may be the right time to do that. There are many different faiths and religions and religion may be the framework for your beliefs or you may adopt a specific philosophy by which you choose to sustain your spiritual energy.

> To forgive is the highest, most beautiful form of love. In return, you will receive untold peace and happiness.
>
> Robert Muller, *Bag of Jewels*

Take a moment to reflect: What is it that sustains your spirit during difficult times?

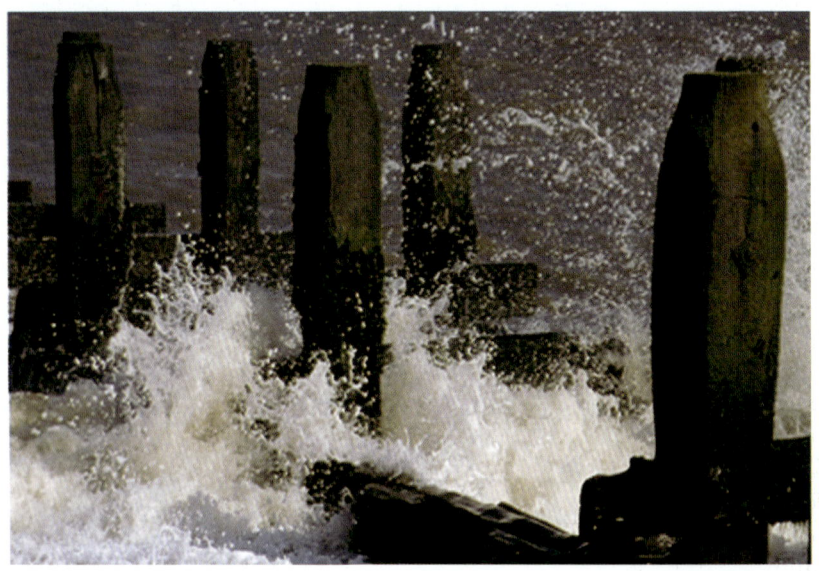

The Soul would have no rainbow, had the eyes no tears.

John Vance Cheney, *Bag of Jewels*

Beliefs and Values

A baby enters this world with a mind, body and spirit in perfect harmony. As it grows its body needs to be nourished, its mind needs to explore and learn through thought processes and behaviour and the spirit needs to be nurtured. As the child grows it develops its own faith, which sustains the spirit.

Faith can be any number of things, such as being a member of an organised religion, adhering to the Ten Commandments, asking for forgiveness and absolution, being a member of Native American Indians, the list is endless. You will find a spiritual path that is right for you, that will nourish you in times of trouble or during a spiritual crisis. But you may decide to ignore your spirit, which will undoubtedly cause imbalance and existential discord.

Many religions are based on a central truth, which is 'God is love'. What would our world be like if we all lived by this truth? Simplistic it maybe; however, it is often the simplest things in life that make a real difference.

As we develop we form our own beliefs and values based on our experience. We assume our culture's beliefs are valid, our moral integrity is appropriate and our values are fulfilling. But as you mature you begin to ask questions and explore new ideas, new religions and different spiritual pathways. Defining spiritual care is difficult because the connection defies translation into words.

Clinical staff, when trying to define spiritual connection with a patient, identified it as often a silent communication conveyed through eye-to-eye contact, where without doubt, spiritual love was shared through the touch of a gentle hand, reaching out to another. Many other clinical staff defined it as a moment captured, as being at one with the world while experiencing:

- a dramatic sunset or sunrise

- a woodland walk, reminding you that we are all part of the universe

- a walk along the shore, allowing you to recognise the power of the sea and how we are just a speck of sand in the greater order of things

Some of the cancer patients also found words inadequate, but felt a connection of unconditional love with the practitioner.

The clinical staff felt that their own spiritual needs were met by support from their own specific beliefs group, organised religion or faith. There is no right or wrong way to sustain your spiritual wellness. It may be a matter of returning to a place of peace and reflection, reconnecting to our world, renewing your faith or a continued searching for your own spiritual pathway.

Patient experience:

> A young woman called Claire in her early forties was experiencing difficulties in arranging appointments for investigations because of her diary commitments. She elected to have the investigations and surgery in the private health sector, as she was financially secure, and had flexability to work around her diary.
>
> Her consultant asked me to see her four weeks after surgery, as she appeared to be really struggling in coming to terms with her cancer and her treatment. When I saw her she was fighting back the tears and I sat her down and began to listen to her.
>
> This determined lady had mapped out her life to achieve the position she had always aspired to. Work was her life. She had always looked after her body, but her mind was stressed and anxious, with periods of obsession and compulsion. She acknowledged that she:

- was determined

- was single-minded

- worked 24/7

- was unable to commit to an intimate relationship

- had given up her social life

- had distanced herself from family and friends

- was financially comfortable

- was very independent

To her, this was who she was. Cancer was not part of her equation. The surgery should have removed the cancer and she should now return to her normal life, centred on her diary.

She had recently been made aware that she would need further treatment and suddenly she felt vulnerable and out of control. Her material wealth was not enough and her ego had priority over her spiritual energy. For the first time in her life she had to ask for help and she found that difficult, as she had always been self-sufficient and did not know how to ask for help.

She wrote to me twelve months later, saying that having cancer had given her a life-changing opportunity, to evaluate her priorities and change her life completely. The first thing she did was to get rid of her diary!

Simplistically, people in times of difficulty usually pray and it often starts with, 'I will do anything, God, if you just help my wife, mother, daughter, son, husband and father through this.' The crisis passes and again God is forgotten. Why is that?

Abbot Christopher, from a UK monastery, wrote a guide for the monk's spiritual practice. His book Finding Sanctuary sets out the monastic steps for everyday life and it is based on seven rules for life:

Silence:

Silences are necessary for finding sanctuary and peace, in a busy and noisy world. Set time aside each day to be still and quiet whether at home, in the garden or in a church.

Contemplation:

Meditating through breathing, prayer or reading is a necessary step to observe daily.

Obedience:

Listening, mutual love and giving up control are the ways that we become true to ourselves and each other.

Humility:

In any human interaction that goes wrong there is usually, somewhere, a lack of humility and an excess of arrogance. Learning how to practise humility is about our struggle to be fully human and about the desire to be rooted in our spiritual self.

Community:

Good conversation, good listening and mutual respect are the foundations of good communities and learning these skills is essential if human beings are to be their best self.

Spirituality:

True spirituality is not picking and mixing or treating the serious things of life as if they were items to be bought from a supermarket. Developing spirituality requires steadfastness and commitment.

Hope:

Finding and living in sanctuary is a lifelong quest. When you fall, which you will, get up and persevere.

There are many faiths and religions, all of which essentially acknowledge the need for unconditional love, to our self and from our self to our neighbours. Religion can be the framework of your beliefs, or the philosophy of your life, or in fact neither of these.

Your spirit encompasses your own beliefs, values and/or life philosophy, which is then able to sustain you in times of trouble or darkness. Having cancer or knowing someone close to you who has cancer may be one of these difficult times.

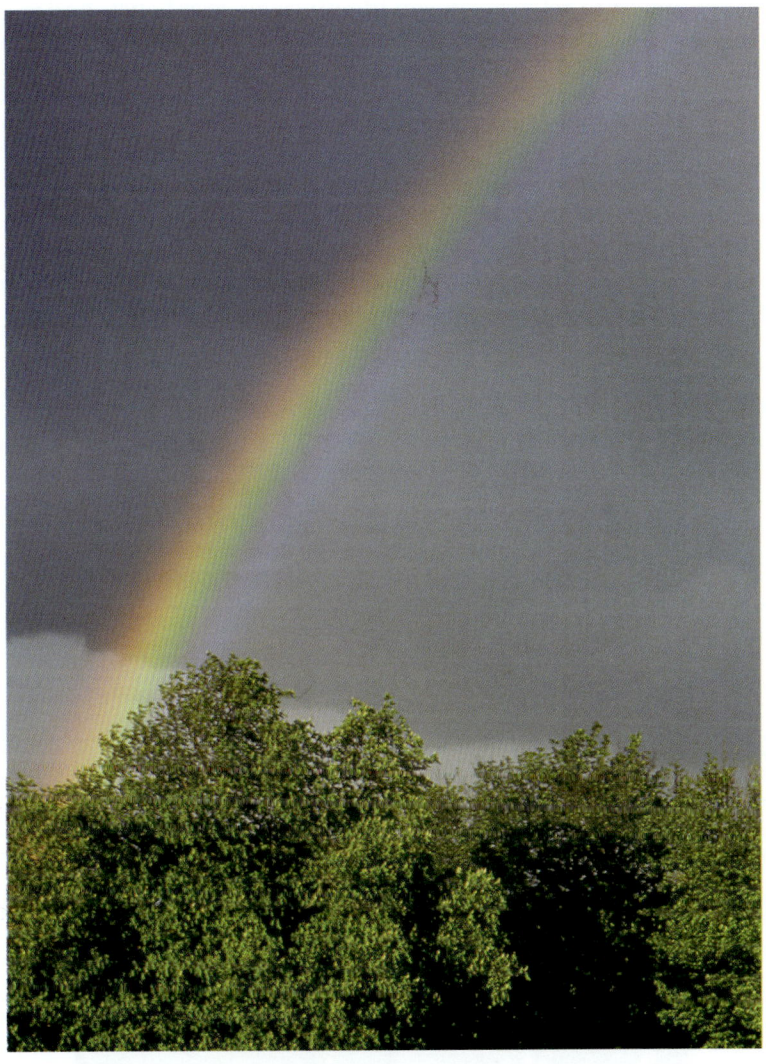

My heart is tuned to the quietness that the stillness of
nature inspires.

Hazrat Inayat Khan, *Taking Time To Just Be*

Take a moment to reflect: can you identify your own beliefs and values? Are your beliefs and values positively supporting you, as you face cancer?

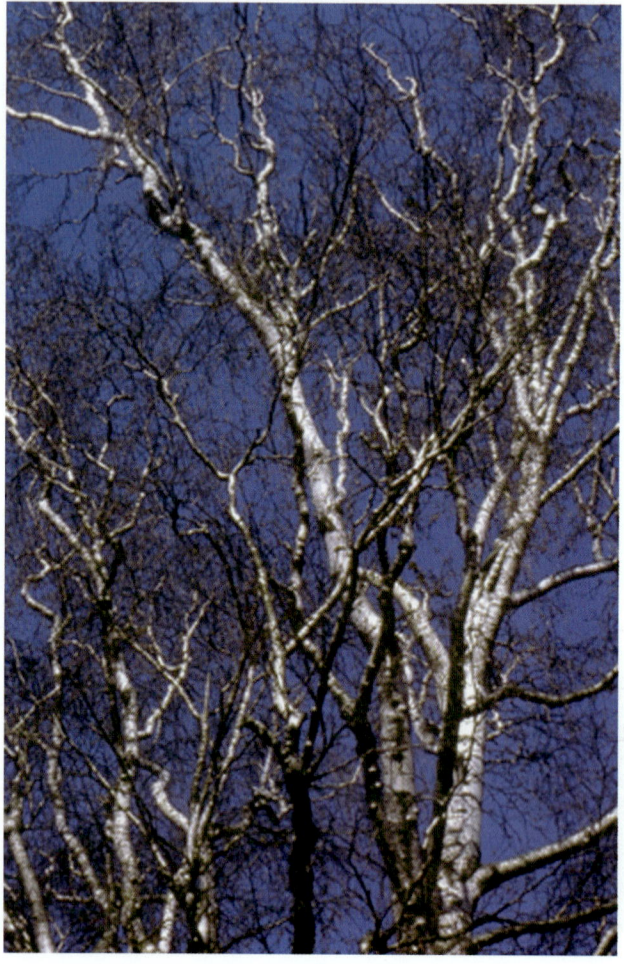

Even if something is left undone, everyone must take time to sit still and watch the leaves turn.

Elizabeth Lawrence, *Take Time To Just Be*

Meditation for the Spirit

Meditation is the process by which we bring the mind into the here and now and it strengthens the spirit against stress. To meditate is to find the presence of true peace. Meditation takes thoughts from the past and the future and returns our mind to the present moment. Through meditation:

- the brain's electrical activity is calmed through an increase in brain waves associated with deep relaxation

- the body's metabolic rate, blood pressure and pulse rate all decrease, allowing more efficient use of oxygen.

- The body's internal healing force is stimulated to produce chemical changes within cells.

Meditation helps us to attain a sense of self and the path to it brings a strong serenity and inner peace that remains strong even in situations of stress.

The physiological effects of meditation if used every day facilitate a greater enthusiasm in everyday life and reduce feelings of anxiety. Meditation is about focusing on doing just one thing at a time. Most of the time we are doing several things at once. Even when you are listening and talking you are also thinking about what you are going to do next. The messages between your mind and your body are constantly altering your energy levels. Do not get frustrated if you find clearing the mind difficult at first. Just acknowledge the thoughts that enter and let them go. The benefits of meditation are well worth your continued persistence. Remember to:

- find a meditation that is right for you

- be patient at first and practise every day

- Initially meditate for up to fifteen minutes a day

- when you are ready you can increase your meditation to twenty to thirty minutes a day

- try to keep the chant or affirmation you are comfortable with for about three to five days before changing it

With practice you will be happy to extend the time each day, giving your mind and body greater benefit. If you feel anxious, just concentrate on your breathing to relax and calm the feeling of anxiety. You may feel bored during meditation. Acknowledge this as resistance to meditation and start to quieten the mind and return to your breathing or mantra. Not everyone will engage with meditation and some may find visualisation easier and more effective for them. Many patients loved the 'changing seasons' visualisation, as for them it was easier to visualise than to clear the mind. Spend some time looking at different types of meditation and visualisation books, to find what is right for you.

> Patient experience:
>
> At the end of a meditation, a patient came and talked to me. She felt she was unable to participate in the meditation, although she had no trouble at home using her own meditation. We explored the specific meditation I had used and realised that its content had been around the sea. The patient admitted that she was afraid of water and because of that, it had ruined her meditation. It is worth remembering to check if the meditation is appropriate for you.

The meditation process:

One of the most important things is to find a place to meditate. It should be a quiet area that is yours and somewhere for you to sit in a position that is comfortable to you, preferably with your feet on the ground and hands resting gently in your lap. If you meditate outside in the summer, some people like to kick off their shoes and make contact with the environment. You may find sitting up straight on a chair is not possible, so in these cases you can either find a chair that is more supportive or rest against pillows on your bed. If you are not comfortable you will find it impossible to maintain your meditation. As you begin to meditate remember the following:

Stillness:

Being able to relax when sitting is important. If you start to fidget or become aware that you are feeling uncomfortable, your meditation will be broken. Maintain stillness through comfort throughout the meditation.

Silence:

Try in the beginning to meditate during a quiet time of your day. If there are other people in the house, let them know you do not want to be disturbed. Turn off the TV, radio, iPod and dwell in the silence. If you can eventually meditate while going around the supermarket, or in a busy airport, you will know you can really meditate.

Sensitivity:

When you begin any new meditation it is helpful to listen, watch and perceive whatever images, symbols, sounds and other sensations appear in your mind. These may be fleeting at first, but by noticing them you will aid the whole process. Your spirit needs quality time in order that you can continue your search for self.

Never waste time and energy wishing you were somewhere else, doing something else. Accept your situation and realize you are where you are, doing what you are doing, for a specific reason. Realise that nothing is by chance, that you have certain lessons to learn and that the situation you are in has been given to you to enable you to learn those lessons as quickly as possible, so that you can move onward and upward along your spiritual path.

Eileen Caddy, *Bag of Jewels*

Take a moment to reflect: what do you feel about meditation? Can you approach it with an open mind?

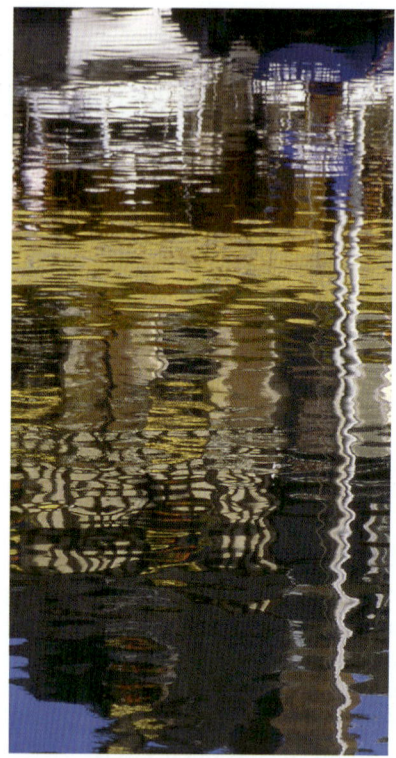 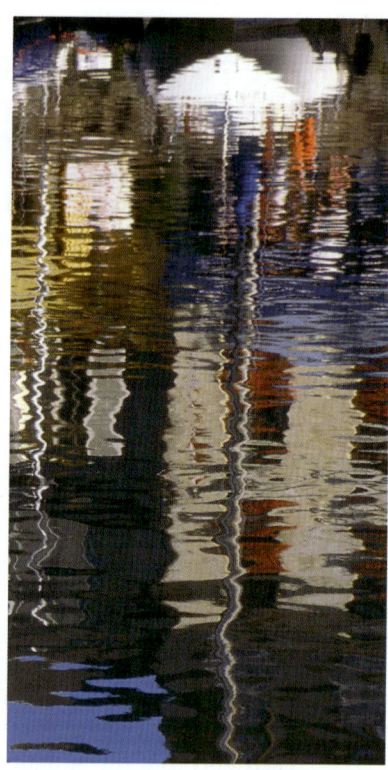

The greatest pleasure in life is doing what people say you cannot do.

Walter Bagehot, *Begin It Now*

Enhancing Intuition

> Trust your intuition – Listen to your intuition – Go with your intuition

Meditation is a way to still the logical mind and bring it under the guidance of higher consciousness. Intuition is defined as quick and ready insight; or the power of attaining direct knowledge without evident rational thought or the drawing of conclusions from evidence. Intuition overshadows the needs and desires of the personal ego. There are several ways of enhancing your intuition:

- dreams are means by which the soul communicates with the conscious mind

- through the arts: painting, sculpture, dance, drama, poetry, storytelling and song

- the newspaper or a TV programme – something you read, watched or listened to which is exactly the experience you needed at that moment in time

Developing the ability to interpret messages from your natural environment enhances your intuition. When you are guided by your intuition, you also open up your creative pathways. Intuition and creativity are very much related; they are the natural resources of the right-hand side of the brain.

> Regret is about:

> If only ...
> I could have ...
> I should have ...
> I would have ...

> Life is far too short for regrets!
> Patricia Gauden

Take a moment to reflect: do you trust your intuition?

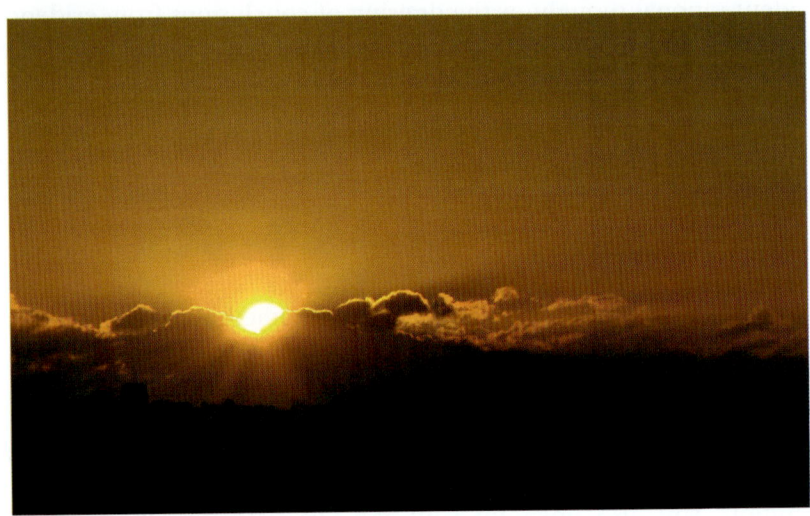

Follow your heart, your dreams, your desires. Do what your soul calls you to do, whatever it is, and allow it to be finished; then you will go on to another adventure.

Ramtha, *Begin it Now*

Spiritual Healing

The spirit is the divine inspiration of the human ensemble. Each and every cell is invested with the energy of the spirit. It is this that fuses the energy of mind and body into one meaning and purpose. The spirit's ability to recognise the sacred presence in all life compels the mind in its striving towards the ideal. Faith, love and surrender allow the energy of the spirit to flow freely. This empowers the essential change needed to bring the energy of body, mind and spirit into perfect balance. Your spiritual energy is based on:

- love, as the breath of life

- My relationship with family, friends and other loved ones, gives me my greatest source of joy

- Feeling goodwill and compassion towards others, rewards me

- Filling your life surrounded by people who care

- Not harbouring resentment towards anyone

- love is the greatest healer of all

- unconditional love being the sign of ultimate wisdom

- the worst kind of poverty being loneliness and feeling unwanted

- I try to infuse my life with love and forgiveness

- I would not purposely hurt any other living thing

- I give kindness with a glad heart to every living creature

- I see beauty in all earth's creatures

- I believe that life is sacred

- I am readily able to apologise, and to accept the apology of other people, and then move on

- I believe it is important to love and respect the elderly

- I beleive that everyone deserves forgiveness; even people who have caused me pain

- I treat others as I would wish to be treated

- I recognise the spirit within me and I feel a sacred presence

- the idea that even-mindedness in all situations is a precious tool

- the fact that life fills me with wonder, amazement and awe

- I believe in my own goodness and inner strength

- I take care of my body as the home of my soul

- truth is essential at all times

- Lifes journey is a glorious adventure

- I often feel overwhelmed by the beauty around me

- the sacredness of life is beyond words

- I believe that surrender is the highest form of freedom

- giving joy to others fills me with happiness

- I believe that material objects bring transient pleasure, but true joy comes from within

- No matter how difficult as things may get, I never give up

- A higher power guides me

- Being kind, compassionate, loving and forgiving, gives me peace of mind

The seeds of healing, at all levels, is about learning to let go. The inner healer is that part of us which knows wholeness and seeks to re-establish this state whenever possible. Embracing the true concept of the inner healer means acknowledging its work on every level: emotional, intellectual, physical and spiritual. Working with our inner healer requires you to take responsibility for our own health and well-being. Listening or tuning in to your spirit is an essential first step in working with and through the inner healer. Remember that it is your own spiritual beliefs and values which govern your response to stress.

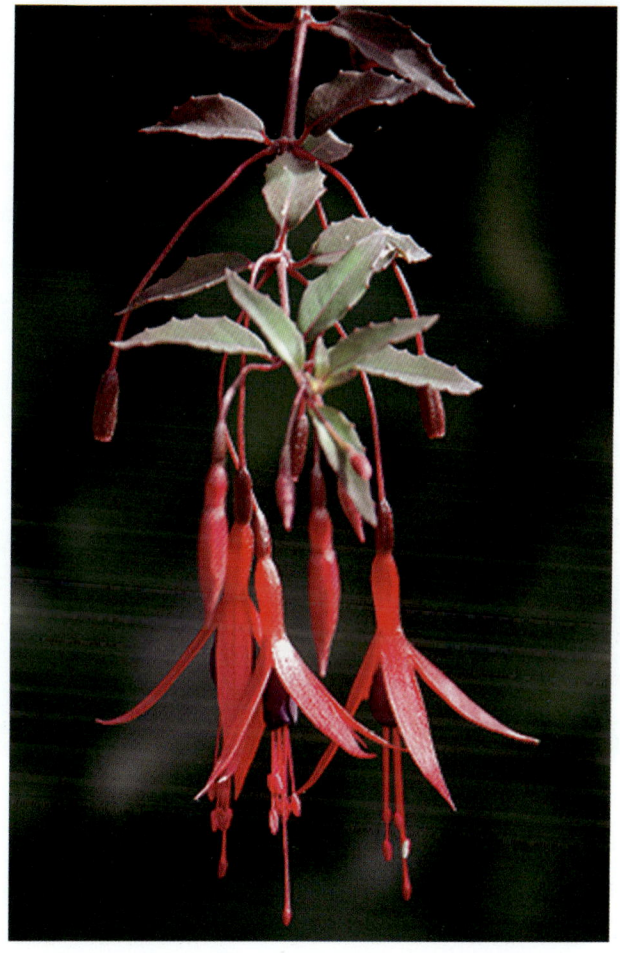

Take a moment to reflect: what does spiritual healing mean to you?

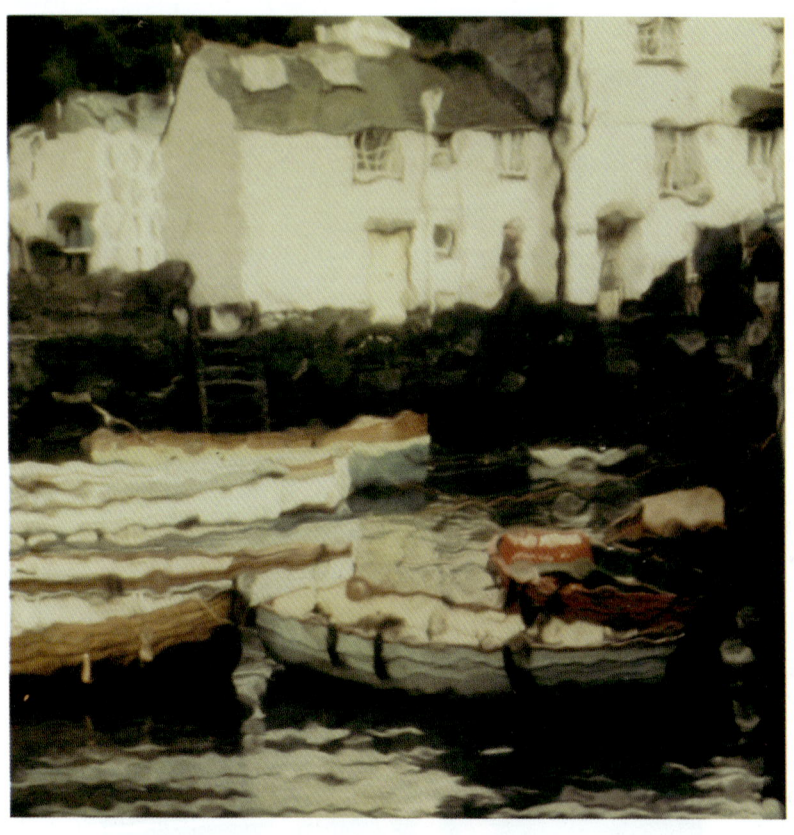

If you are losing your leisure, look out; you may be losing your soul.

Logan Pearsall Smith, *Taking Time To Just Be*

Rediscover your Creativity, Ambitions and Lost Dreams

> If you are seeking creative dreams, go out walking. Angels
> whisper to a man when he goes for a walk.
>
> Raymond Inmon (*Bag of Jewels*)

When did you last put on your wellington boots and walk through
puddles in the rain, or walk along a seashore at dusk, watching the sun
go down? Somehow, life has become too busy, trying to fit everything
in and cope with the cancer as well. One thing is for sure, the washing,
ironing, cleaning and shopping will still need doing tomorrow, next
week, next month, so why not act spontaneously and make time
for you!

What is it you have always wanted to do but always put off? Have you
wanted to explore new areas of creativity but somehow putting time
aside for you seemed too hard to achieve each day? On the days you are
recovering from your treatment, take some time to plan all that you
want to achieve! The longer you put things off, the more likely it is that
you will never achieve them. Remember the saying 'Don't put off till
tomorrow what can be done today'.

During your treatment and recovery from cancer make time count.
Why not start a scrapbook, put yourself in the picture and then around
you put all the things you have wanted to do. Use any art or craft
materials you have: drawings, pictures from magazines, postcards,
poems, words, photographs, etc. On another page of the scrapbook,
show how you would celebrate finishing your treatment or being
disease free for one year. You may have lost all hope of going on that
special holiday or seeing a loved one who lives on the other side of the
world. Construct that picture and renew your ambitions or dreams, as
only you can, and then set your goal to make it happen.

It is helpful to create a different page in your scrapbook for specific
events you have achieved in your life, so it does not become too
complex. Treat yourself to a beautiful memory box or create your own
and in it put pictures, photos and keepsakes from the magical moments
you have had in your life. Remember to:

- depict the situation in its complete form as if it already exists

- avoid showing anything negative or undesirable

- aim to use lots of colour

- make it look achievable

- include a symbol of your spirit energy, which has meaning and purpose for you

- put in some positive affirmations

- spend a few minutes each day quietly looking at the pages you have created!

A scrapbook is visual and easy to refer to each day. It also allows you to share what you want to achieve with your friends and family. Another way of achieving your ambitions and dreams is to positively plan for them. If you want to realise them, then think about when you want them to happen and what steps you have to take to achieve them. Write down your goals for the next week, the next month, the next six months, the next year. Choose your own time frame. Some examples include:

- be healthy

- take up art

- learn a new skill

- move house

- write a book

- visit a special part of the world

- give up worrying!

- ride in a hot-air balloon

- horse-ride along the beach at sunset

- give yourself a treat every day, or week

- take that cruise you have always dreamed of

- throw a party, to celebrate your life

- reconnect with your mind, body and spirit

- become a lady who lunches

- take up a new hobby

- go to the opera or the theatre

Choose your own goals and remember that they may change, in which case choose again. Only you can make different choices and change your life. Listen to your intuition, let your mind, body and spirit be your guide and make your lost ambitions and dreams come true!

Patient experience:

During my cancer treatment I had time to begin to rediscover my creativity. I have always enjoyed the arts, but had not really done anything creative for over ten years. Whilst recovering from chemotherapy I decided that I wanted to portray my life through art, as three separate projects:

Project one:

A scrapbook for my daughter showing my life up until she was born, my life as a child and a teenager, my first love, my wedding day, my job and hobbies.

Project two:

I wanted to depict, through a series of watercolour paintings, my experience of being told I had cancer, undergoing treatment and living with cancer after treatment had finished.

Project three:

I wanted to tell the story of our life together as a family, so that we all could have input into this project, which would be ongoing until my daughter married.

Part of the reason for wanting to do this was to validate my life and the things I have done at all stages of my life. I have finished the first project, the scrapbook, the paintings are ongoing and as a family we have started the photo project. It has been a wonderful experience and very cathartic for me. I feel alive again!

Many patients viewed the scrapbook as a positive achievement. It was also about having fun with family and friends. 'I felt alive and connected to those around me,' she said. It is about taking the life-changing opportunity of cancer to reconnect with yourself and others. The choice is now yours; will you take this life-changing opportunity? For you can now assess your mind, body and spirit's energy, and how to balance it ...

Take a moment to reflect: cancer is limited; it cannot:

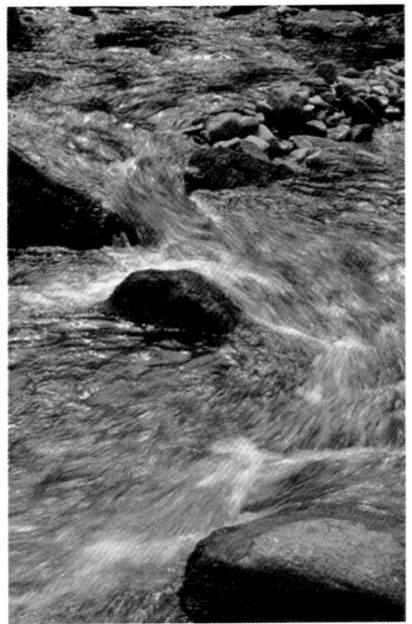

- Cripple love
- Shatter hope
- Corrode faith
- Eliminate peace
- Destroy confidence
- Kill friendship
- Obliterate memories
- Silence courage
- Invade your soul.

Appendix I

Art Therapy

For art therapy you do not have to spend money on equipment. You can use any medium you like: finger paints, watercolour paints, coloured pencils, poster paint, etc. Likewise, you only need one paintbrush. You can use any paper, just something you have lying around, and some old magazines are perfect, along with an old shoebox, glue and a scrapbook.

Shoebox exercise:

This exercise can be fun, especially if you do it within a group; though it can also be done when you are on your own. You will need magazines, glue and an old shoebox. The objective is to honestly look at who you are on the outside, you in your various roles, the person you are happy for others to see. Cover the outside of the box with all these pictures. When finished on the outside, start on the inside. Fill the box or stick pictures inside the box of who you really are. The person that maybe only you or those close to you know. The outcome is to see if there is a difference between the two and to try to bring more of what is on the inside to the outside!

The picture before, now and after the patient receiving radiotherapy: This technique can be used when you are having to face something that you would rather not. Choose a magazine and in it choose a picture. When you get to the appointment, or whilst at the actual event, look at the picture and in your head create a story of what was going on before the picture was taken. Recall the picture or change it, and after the event put your own ending on the story. This is a useful experience when facing anything that you are not comfortable with such as treatment.

Create your own story:

You can use music or a poem for this. Listen to the music or read the poem and then paint what it was saying to you; paint how you feel. How did the music or poem change your emotions? How did it make you feel? It is important that you choose something that you like for this exercise.

Another way to express what you are feeling is to just sit down and without thought, just paint. Don't think about it, just go with the music. When the music stops, look at the picture and try to explain what it is about. What are the colours you have used? Is the picture happy or sad?

Then try listening to a favourite cd and go back to your painting, turn over the page and paint what you are now feeling. Can you see a difference in the two pictures?

You do not have to be an artist – you don't have to let anyone see what you have done; only you will know what works for you!

Appendix II

Music Therapy – engage with life

Fighting-spirit music:

When you want to push forward with all your fighting spirit, use a piece of music that to you emphasises just that. It may help to visualise your body's immune system fighting to return to normal, or your cells slaying the malignant cells. Playing the music on the way to the hospital for treatment is a good time to do this.

Many cancer patients felt that once diagnosed, the normal things in their everyday life changed. Somehow, life became more serious and the noise of the everyday radio or music fell silent.

Mood music:

Music can set the mood for many aspects of your life. Spend an afternoon looking at your music collection and identify what mood each cd would set. Do you have music to move to? Music to relax you, fire you up or make you laugh or cry? Do you have any music with special memories or something you can meditate to?

These days, music is all around us and today's culture of iPods and MP3 players allows you to readily download specific music for different occasions. Use headphones that can block out everyday sounds, allowing you to remain in your personal space.

On days that are difficult for you to express what you feel, put on a cd or track, close your eyes and listen to the music. At the end, write or paint what emotions you were feeling whilst listening to it. Has your mood changed?

When you have a moment, close your eyes and think about now, today, and what you are feeling. Are you sad, lonely, angry, frustrated, isolated, fearful or anxious? These are all negative emotions. When you open your eyes, write down the emotion you are feeling.

Would a loved one know from your poem or drawing what you were feeling? Turn the page over and write or draw how you feel using a positive emotion. When you have finished compare the two. Which one would you like to feel? It is up to you to make it happen. We all put on a face for other people, but how much pain does this cause you by not being true to yourself?

Therapeutic writing:

Meet up with a friend or family member for lunch and whilst there, write a paragraph describing yourself. Also ask the person with whom you are having lunch to write a paragraph describing you. Then compare and share each other's thoughts.

Another example is to write on one side of the paper five things that you like and on the opposite side five things you dislike. Do your family and friends know what you like or dislike? Do they know:

what makes you happy?

what makes you laugh?

what hurts you?

what makes you angry?

who your friends are?

what your home is like?

what your hopes are?

what you dream of?

Is it that you do not want others to see who you really are? Do you find it difficult to share information about yourself with others?

Why not ring some friends or close family and invite them around for afternoon tea? You could arrange for a face painter to be there and have your face painted as an animal, and then act out the animal you are. It is great to just laugh and have fun; children do it, so why not you? Why not meet up with friends every so often, get some popcorn and chocolate, and watch a film. For an hour or so, forget who you are and have fun – you deserve it!

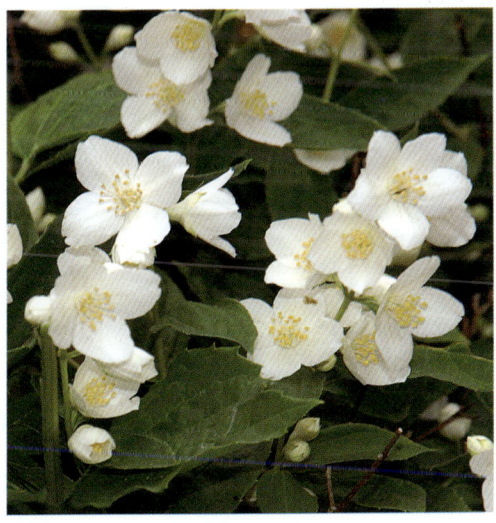

Patient experience:

There are now many patients who live on their own, some of whom do not have family and friends close by. One such patient, Jane, decided after reading *Bridget Jones' Diary* that she would keep a diary for a year and instead of noting how much she weighed each day, and how much alcohol she'd had, she would record one thing her body was doing each day, and one thing her mind was telling her each day. She wanted to keep a diary of her treatment and this seemed a fun way to do it. She decided that if there were more entries in the diary that were positive, she would reward herself at the end of the year with a special spa weekend. If the diary had more negative entries she would find a suitable punishment for the end of the year!

At the end of the year, she was astonished at the number of funny moments that had happened. At one of her group sessions at a cancer centre, she read sections of her diary to the other patients and it was an enormous success, and was enjoyed by everyone. She now has friends locally and has found that having cancer really did give her a life-changing opportunity.

Further Reading

Chopra, Deepak, *Grow Younger, Live Longer: Ten Steps to Reverse Aging* (Rider, 2001)

Dossey, Larry, MD, *Meaning & Medicine: Lessons from a Doctor's Tales of Breakthrough and Healing* (Bantam, 1992)

Dyer, Wayne W., *There is a Spiritual Solution to Every Problem* (HarperCollins, 2002)

Einstein, Patricia, *Intuition: The Path to Inner Wisdom* (Element Books Inc. 1997)

Hay, Louise, *You Can Heal Your Life* (Santa Monica, Hay House, 1984)

Lawless, Julia, *Encyclopaedia of Essential Oils: A Complete Guide to the Use of Aromatic Oils in Aromatherapy, Herbalism, Health and Well-being* (Element Books, 1992)

LeShan, Lawrence, *You Can Fight For Your Life* (Thorsons, 1984)

Levin, Michael, *Spiritual Intelligence: awakening the power of your spirituality and intuition* (London, Hodder and Stoughton, 2000)

Levin, Michael, *Meditation: Path to the Deepest Self* (Dorling Kindersley Limited, 2002)0

Pert, Candace B., *Molecules of Emotion: the Science Behind Mind–Body Medicine* (Simon and Schuster Inc. 1997)

Reynolds, Caroline, *Spiritual Fitness* (Thorsons; an imprint of HarperCollins Publishers, 2001)

Shapiro, Eddie and Shapiro, Debbie, *Meditation of Inner Peace: your guide to relaxation and true happiness* (Judy Piatkus Publishers Ltd, 1997)

Shaw, Claire, *The Power of Food: Cancer – Food, Facts & Recipes* (Octopus Publishing Group Ltd, 2005)

Siegel, Bernie, *Love, Medicine and Miracles* (New York, HarperCollins, 1986)

Simon, David, *Return to Wholeness: Embracing Body, Mind and Spirit in the Face of Cancer* (John Wiley and Sons Inc. 1999)

Simonton, O. C., S. Matthews-Simonton and J. Creighton, *Getting Well Again* (Los Angeles, J. P. Tarcher, 1978)

Vaughan, Frances and Walsh, Roger, A *Course in Miracles: Accept This Gift* (Jeremy P. Tarcher Inc. Foundation for Inner Peace, 1983)

Walsh, Roger, *Essential Spirituality: The 7 Central Practices to Awaken the Heart and Mind* (John Wiley and Sons Inc. 1999)

Weil, Andrew, *Spontaneous Healing: How to Discover and Enhance your Body's Ability to Maintain and Heal Itself* (New York, Knopf, 1995)

Wright, S. G. and Sayre-Adams, Jean, *Sacred Space: Right Relationship and Spirituality in Healthcare* (Harcourt Publishers Ltd, 2000)

Zukav, Gary, *The Seat of the Soul* (St Martin's Press, 1990)

Acknowledgements

Billingsley, Jim, *Reflections: A Calligraphic Journey Through the Wisdom of Words* (UK, Selecta Books Ltd, 1993)

Brown, Pam, McFarland, Stuart and Linda, *Taking Time Just To Be*, Helen Exley (ed.) (2005) [website] <http://www.helenexleygiftbooks> (accessed 2003)

Hayward, Susan, and Cohan, Malcolm, *Bag of Jewels* (AU, In-Tune Books, 1987)

Hayward, Susan, *Begin It Now: You Have A Purpose* (AU, In-Tune Books, 1987)

Whilst every effort has been made to trace copyright holders, the publishers would be pleased to hear from any not here acknowledged.

Support Agencies

American Association of Music Therapy [website] <http://www.musictherapy.org>

Breakthrough Breast Cancer, Registered Office, 3rd Floor Weston House, 246 High Holborn, London WC1V 7EX [website] <http://www.breakthrough.org.uk>

Breast Cancer Care, 5-13 Great Suffolk Street, London, SE1 0NS

Breast Cancer Care Helpline (Tel: 0808 800 6000; [website] <http://www.breastcancercare.org.uk>)
Breast Cancer Care – Scotland (Tel: 0845 077 1892)
Breast Cancer Care – Wales (Tel: 0845 077 1894)
Breast Cancer Care – North & Midlands (Tel: 0845 077 1893)
Breast Cancer Care – London & South (Tel: 0845 077 1895)
Breast Cancer Care Central Office, 5–13 Great Suffolk Street, London SE1 0NS (Tel: 020 7384 2984)

Cancer BACUP, 3 Bath Place, Rivington Street, London EC2A 3JR. (Tel: 020 7696 9003) (Freephone Macmillan Cancer Support Helpline: 0808 808 0000) Cancer BACUP is the UK's leading cancer information charity (Freephone Helpline: 0808 800 1234 Monday–Friday 9.00 a.m.–8.00 p.m. Cancer BACUP provide over 70 booklets and over 300 fact sheets dealing with each type of cancer and its treatment [website] <http://www.cancerbackup.org.uk>

CancerLine (Tel: 0808 808 2020) [website] <http://www.macmillan.org.uk>

Institute for Complementary Medicine (ICM), PO Box 194, London SE16 7QZ (Tel: 020 7237 5165)

International Federation of Aromatherapists, Stanford House, 2–4 Chiswick High Road, London W4 1TH (Tel: 0181 742 2605/6)

Macmillan Cancer Support, 89 Albert Embankment, London SE1 7UQ (Tel: 020 7840 7840)
Cancerline: (0808 808 2020)

Marie Curie Cancer Care, 89 Albert Embankment, London SE1 7TP (Tel: 020 7599 7777) www.mariecurie.org.uk

Penny Brohn Cancer Care (formerly Bristol Cancer Help Centre), Chapel Pill Lane, Pill, Bristol BS20 0HH (Helpline: 0845 123 23 10) [website] <http://www.pennybrohncancercare.org>

The British Holistic Medical Association, Trust House, Royal Shrewsbury Hospital, South Shropshire SY3 8XF (Tel: 01743 261155)

The Register of Qualified Aromatherapists, PO Box 6941, London N8 9HF (Tel: 0208341 2958)